Mediterranean Diet for Beginners 2020

The Complete Guide Solutions with Meal Plan and Recipes for Weight Loss, Prevention of Cardiovascular Diseases, Boost your Energy, Reset Your Body Living Healthier and Longer

Elizabeth Ryan

Copyright © 2020 by Elizabeth Ryan

means or in printed format. Recording of this publication is strictly prohibited and any storage of this document is not allowed unless with written permission from the publisher.

The information provided herein is stated to be truthful and consistent, in that any liability, in terms of inattention or otherwise, by any usage or abuse of any policies, processes, or directions contained within is the solitary and utter responsibility of the recipient reader.

Under no circumstances will any legal responsibility or blame be held against the publisher for any reparation, damages, or monetary loss due to the information herein, either directly or indirectly. Respective authors own all copyrights not held by the publisher.

The information herein is offered for informational purposes solely, and is universal as so.

The presentation of the information is without contract or any type of guarantee assurance.

The trademarks that are used are without any consent, and the publication of the trademark is without permission or backing by the trademark owner.

All trademarks and brands within this book are for clarifying purposes only and are the owned by the owners themselves, not affiliated with this document.

Contents

WHAT IS MEDITERRANEAN DIET

Mediterranean diet is a method for eating dependent on conventional foods and eating examples of the individuals and nations encompassing the Mediterranean Sea.

The Mediterranean Diet isn't a diet. It is a deep-rooted propensity. Something you should adhere to as an ideology. Decades prior, this was the standard lifestyle of the networks around the Mediterranean Basin. It was the regular day to day existence in nations like Spain, Italy or Greece. Its significant focuses were physical movement, healthy sustenance, and quiet demeanor. And very little cash to discard.

These components molded the Mediterranean culture. It is the main diet to have been granted this acknowledgment.

These days, the outside impact has changed the first propensities in those nations. Many qualified individuals are endeavoring to get back what is the best nourishment design on the planet.

The Mediterranean Diet is an ideal approach to live for numerous years. And to live them well. It will keep you fit as a fiddle, keep up your skin perfect and wonderful, and make your organs work appropriately.

It is the correct diet to keep you on the shape, without dangers.

Along these lines, kindly, don't imperil your wellbeing with earnest and lopsided lack of healthy sustenance.

The Mediterranean diet concentrates more on fruits, veggies, whole grains, beans, nuts, and legumes (base of the pyramid); lean proteins from fish and poultry; great fats from olive oil; and some dairy–while devouring desserts and red meats on fewer events (top of the pyramid)

The Mediterranean diet isn't a "diet" essentially. It is a blend of the conventional eating propensities for individuals living in Spain, Italy, France, Greece, and the Middle East.

Is the Mediterranean Diet costly?

There is something you ought to consider. The Mediterranean Diet is free, without any enhancements or packs. There aren't any financial interests behind it. The leading cash you will spend is the one you put resources into crisp food, fruits, and vegetables.

What can it accomplish for you?

The Mediterranean Diet is an ideal approach to forestall numerous diseases. The fundamental is the stroke and respiratory failure. It likewise prevents metabolic syndrome, lung diseases, asthma, allergies, Parkinson's, Alzheimer's, and decalcification.

It keeps the bone mass in old individuals. And it is connected to low occurrences of numerous sorts of malignant growth.

The Mediterranean Diet can keep you healthy and glad.

The first Mediterranean Diet qualities are:

1. High utilization of virgin olive oil.

2. High admission of vegetables and fruits and legumes.

3. Use of non-refined starches (segments to be changed in accordance with physical action).

4. Consumption of fish, particularly slick (or "somewhat blue" one) three or four times each week

5. Consumption of milk, cheddar, and yogurt. The first cheddar was a new goat cheddar). Watch out for the soaked fats of the dairy items.

6. Three or four eggs for each week.

7. Moderate utilization of meat and soaked fats (common, not misleadingly hydrogenated!).

8. One or two little glasses of wine a day, at the primary dinners. White wine and brew are choices.

9. Nuts as tidbits. In "unique events" Mediterranean Diet conventional treats.

10. Do physical exercise!

If you need to diminish your weight, you should pick the fewer caloric supplements. Or on the other hand, simply do the inverse to build it.

In the event that you need to diminish your weight, you should pick the fewer caloric supplements. Or on the other hand, simply do the inverse to expand it.

Mediterranean Diet devotees have a 70% greater amount of hope of life. An 80% of better quality life, assuming they don't smoke. In the event that you search for a healthy life, what is the utilization of smoking?

What to pick and what to dodge

Adhering to the Mediterranean Diet implies not just picking the correct food. It is progressively critical to maintaining a strategic distance from others.

You need to boycott all the business and fake items. They didn't exist fifty or sixty years prior. They are misleadingly hydrogenated items and subsidiaries, and anything associated with containing trans-fats. In the USA, it is mandatory in January. First, 2006 to appear in the names of the trans-fat extent. You ought to pick items with 0% of trans fats. You ought to think about that 0% implies right up to 0.49 grams per serving. In the event that the serving is little and you take many, you may eat a ton of these fats. They increment the terrible cholesterol (LDL) and diminish the great one (HDL). Aside from other guessed negative impacts.

Avoid prevailing fashion diets! They may demolish your wellbeing.

Individuals learn the Mediterranean Diet early and in a characteristic manner. Guardians need to encourage their youngster's food propensities. Instruct them to maintain a strategic distance from fabricated items. Cause them to pick new and normal food.

Give them an apple, a banana, or a natively constructed sandwich. Keep away from non-normal items. Be cautious with the primary dinners and direct the school's snacks. It is of the most extreme significance. Recollect that your body and cerebrum age will rely upon what you eat!

How to Start the Mediterranean Diet

1. Eat normal, natural foods like fruits, vegetables, whole grains, and nuts.

2. Make olive oil your essential wellspring of dietary fat

3. Reduce the utilization of red meat (Monthly)

4. Eat low to direct measures of fish (Weekly)

5. Drink a moderate measure of wine (up to one to two glasses for every day for men and up to one glass for each day for women)

MEDITERRANEAN DIET GUIDELINES

Unique Mediterranean Diet rules of activity:

1. Make the virgin olive oil your novel fat. Try not to reuse the oil in the wake of singing. We don't suggest profound fryers, yet on the off chance that you need to utilize a less expensive oil for one of these gadgets, purchase high oleic sunflower oil. This oil is a cutting edge fat produced using hereditarily adjusted sunflower seed. It has a piece like virgin olive oil and is as steady as it at high temperatures. It is more extravagant in oleic corrosive than ordinary sunflower oil

Oleic corrosive is a sort of monounsaturated fat quality of olive oil, olives, and avocado, and after this oddity of food innovation, it additionally possesses large amounts of this new kind of oil.

In olive oil, oleic corrosive is available in a proportion of around 70-75%. In the "high oleic" sunflower, around 80%. In avocado, it is to an extent near 70%, while in the regular sunflower oil, this unsaturated fat arrives at just 31.5%.

Oleic corrosive expedites a useful activity in our veins and heart. It expands the "great cholesterol" (HDL-c), adding to diminish the danger of cardiovascular diseases.

Never use shortening for profound broiling. It is an unadulterated trans-fat.

Recall that the fat you put in your life will exacerbate it better or, shorter or more. Put resources into virgin olive oil or in additional virgin olive oil! Basic olive oil is a totally unique item. It is a refined one without the properties of the virgin.

2. Consume loads of vegetables, fruits, and legumes.

3. Buy non-refined starches, genuine whole grain bread, in amounts changed in accordance with your physical movement.

4. Eat much of the time fish, particularly little and slick (or "pale blue" one) three or four times each week.

5. Take every day some dairy items milk and subordinates, cheddar, and yogurt (the first cheddar was crisp goat cheddar). In the event that you are partial to them or are overweight, go for the skimmed forms.

6. Have three or four eggs every week.

7. Take the meat and immersed fats in diminished amounts. Keep away from misleadingly hydrogenated fats at any expense. This way, to evade the fabricated items or to peruse their names cautiously. In the event

that they don't have trans fats, they may have part of sugar.

8. Take a couple of little glasses of wine a day, at the fundamental dinners. White wine and brew are options. Boycott soft drinks and natural product juices.

9. Take nuts and dried fruits as bites and pastries. Watch the calories. In "extraordinary events" have natively constructed Mediterranean Diet conventional sweets.

10. Do physical exercise!

In the event that you pursue these Mediterranean Diet Guidelines, you will have a more beneficial and better life.

Who ought to pursue the Mediterranean diet?

The response to the inquiry, "Who ought to pursue the Mediterranean diet?" is Everyone. Everyone ought to pursue a healthy diet with the goal that the individual in question would be healthy in the body and at the top of the priority list. You ought to recollect that you don't pursue a diet since it is a style or in light of the fact that you need to lose a few pounds quickly. You pursue a diet since you need to have a healthy living. A diet is a method for living, and the Mediterranean diet has been such a diet. It has been the method for living for many individuals in the Mediterranean Sea, and this sort of living has been "found" as of late by dieticians and nutritionists around the globe, who presently urge individuals to tail it.

Is the Mediterranean diet increasingly appropriate for specific individuals? The appropriate response is No.

Mediterranean diet is for all individuals, everything being equal, races, and nationalities. It is as healthy for a white lady in Canada with respect to a Chinese man in Australia. Following the Mediterranean diet, we get security from the sun, we get shielded from malignant growth, and it causes us to battle diabetes and other constant diseases. Mediterranean diet is additionally great and is suitable for Vegetarians. A prescription diet isn't an artificial diet. It is a diet that has developed during that time, so it would serve the preferences and necessities of the countries in the Mediterranean Sea.

Women ought to pursue the Mediterranean diet. Why? An ongoing Harvard study indicated that women who have embraced the Mediterranean diet and method for living, live more, and without disease! The investigation pursued the dietary propensities for around 10 thousand women who were in their fifties and sixties, 50s and 60s for a long time. The outcomes were astounding! Women, who pursued the

Mediterranean diet, eating bunches of fruits and vegetables and other Mediterranean food, were bound to arrive at their 70s healthy and free of ceaseless diseases like heart diseases and diabetes. The rates and proportions were agreeable to the Med diet, and this is nothing unexpected to the vast majority of us, and it is absolutely another bit of persuading information and supporting information in our endeavors to persuade the unconvinced!

In the event that you need to beat Dementia later on in your life, you ought to pursue the Mediterranean diet as right on time as conceivable in your life, since Mediterranean foods are wealthy in omega-3 unsaturated fats which assist us with battling memory and intellectual decrease. It was discovered that individuals who pursue the Mediterranean diet are by 19% less inclined to create thinking and memory issues than individuals who were on some other diet. These outcomes demonstrated again that a healthy diet is a healthy diet regardless of what you look like at it.

Is it true that you are fat? Is it norm to say that you are overweight? Well, the Mediterranean diet is unquestionably for you. Following the Mediterranean diet won't immediately affect your weight. Anyway, you will get in shape step by step, which is the correct method to do it, in a healthy route and in a way which will turn out to be a piece of your life. So individuals who are overweight or experience the ill effects of corpulence should pursue the Mediterraneandiet book "The Mediterranean diet" wherein she clarifies how you can join basic Greek eating propensities and deceives in your diet with the goal that you can make it more advantageous and more delicious! You may attempt it.

Do you like yogurt? Do you love Greek Yogurt? On the off chance that the appropriate response is true, at that point, you are prepared to pursue and embrace the Mediterranean diet. Greek Yogurt is a piece of the Mediterranean diet alongside other dairy items, for example, white cheddar, and you can appreciate them with some restraint. The benefits and nourishing qualities of Greek yogurt are notable, and this is the reason it has gotten so well known in the USA, and it is presently its prominence is expanding in different nations like UK, Canada, and Australia. Greek yogurt is stressed yogurt with substantially more supplements and considerably fewer calories than the typical yogurt.

Will low pay individuals embrace the Mediterranean diet? Off-kilter! Mediterranean diet is neither for the rich nor for the city individuals. It is for everybody. Actually, individuals in the towns of Spain, Greece, Italy, Morocco, and Lebanon are not the most extravagant individuals in their nations, yet they have been living on the Mediterranean diet for thousands of years. You can pick fruits and vegetables which are in season to make your suppers. On the off chance that you can, you can even develop your own vegetables and fruits. Legumes that can be expended consistently are not so costly, and there are numerous scrumptious Mediterranean diet recipes that you can use to make delicious and healthy foods.

The whole family ought to pursue the Mediterranean Diet. This is the response to the inquiry with respect to who ought to pursue the Mediterranean diet. It is imperative to understand that on the off chance that you are a mother or a dad you would need your children to embrace a healthy diet the most punctual in their lives with the goal that they would get familiar with the lifestyle a healthy diet would direct and the sooner they overlook the quick and shoddy nourishment others eat the better it would be for you and their wellbeing. You can supplant unhealthy snacks with a healthy yogurt or a few sticks of carrot or celery, and you can surely diminish the high utilization of red meat and burgers with more advantageous foods like fish, chicken, legumes, and white cheddar. In one of our ongoing articles, "How the whole family can receive the Mediterranean Diet?" we have given some supportive tips for the moms and fathers who need to have a healthy family.

Taking everything into account, we can obviously express that everybody ought to and must pursue the Mediterranean diet. We owe this to ourselves, our families, and our networks. We generally state the aversion is superior to anything fix, and this is the thing that you will do with the Mediterranean diet. By embracing the Med diet, we remain more beneficial, and consequently, we can live more years healthy pushing the incessant diseases further down and presumably maintaining a strategic distance from the majority of them. It ought to be noted here that the Mediterranean diet itself can't make marvels. We have to practice since physical exercise is the second and fundamental piece of a healthy life. You can without much of a stretch exercise by basically strolling 30-40 minutes every day, and this would empower you to be fit. To consolidate the healthy Mediterranean diet with physical exercise, and you will live numerous and healthy years.

MEDITERRANEAN DIET LIFESTYLE

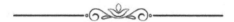

One thing to remember: this isn't a specialist assessment nor an extensive investigation of the Mediterranean lifestyle. This is me, a Mediterranean young lady, sharing my very own point of view on a lifestyle I practice. And I am deciding to share just five things to enable you to understand, and maybe start to pursue the Mediterranean lifestyle. For the absence of an increasingly inventive title, we should go with "5 fundamentals of the Mediterranean lifestyle."

5 Basics of the Mediterranean Lifestyle

Pursue the Mediterranean Diet

Growing up, crisp vegetables, a handful of crude nuts, or even a bowl of lentil soup were my standard after-school snacks. Two times each week, my family ate fish or seafood for supper, frequently with a side of rice or grains and a crisp slashed salad. We ate different types of lean protein like poultry, decently. Red meats now and again. I would lie on the off chance that I said chocolate, cakes, and baked goods never showed up, I mean hi baklava! Be that as it may, a bit of crisp natural product or dried organic product was an increasingly standard pastry decision.

With all the assortment on the Mediterranean food pyramid, it's extremely difficult to believe that my family is following a "diet," correct? There are no food limitations in the Mediterranean diet. Everything is practically permitted.

In any case, on the off chance that you take a gander at the Mediterranean food pyramid, you'll rapidly see that it centers around grains and vegetables; dairy; fiber and lean proteins from nuts and seafood, and far less on greasy meats. Olive oil is additionally a fundamental wellspring of fat (pretty much every formula here on the blog has olive oil as a fixing). And truly, thank heavens, we can have a little wine!

We can positively devote another whole post to the Mediterranean diet alone. However, the key is in adjusting your suppers as indicated by the Mediterranean food pyramid. Eat a greater amount of what's at the wide base of the pyramid; less and less of the things toward the highest point of the pyramid. Obviously, focus on partition sizes; there is no "supersize suppers" in the Mediterranean lifestyle.

Be with family. Offer with friends and family

With regards to eating and bit size, one accommodating Mediterranean propensity is to eat as hardly any dinners as conceivable alone. I grew up eating every one of my suppers at a table brimming with loved ones, and I attempt to do a similar today. I don't think about you; however, when I share a feast with others, I will, in general, eat gradually, and I am less inclined to stuff myself.

Be that as it may, past sharing a feast, the Mediterranean culture develops a reasonable public activity and a specific connectedness to the individuals who matter.

Five years back, when we lived in Iowa, I chose to restrict my public activity. Sounds conflicting, correct? I returned to something I picked up experiencing childhood with the shores of the Mediterranean. Something you may perceive as antiquated Biblical knowledge, "a man with an excessive number of companions, goes to his own ruin." I encircle myself with my family and just a couple of steadfast companions. I encircle myself with individuals who care profoundly about me, individuals that will come clean with me and help me develop. My social schedule liberated.

Move Naturally

Here is a major admission from a genuine Mediterranean lady: Mediterranean people don't work out. I understand that I'm making major speculation, and I realize it appears to be somewhat of an incomprehensible thing to include here. In any case, truly, Mediterranean individuals don't explicitly cut out two hours per day for hard work at the exercise center. In any case, that doesn't make them idle.

Nothing is too advantageous when you live in that piece of the world, so moving is a characteristic practice for individuals of the Mediterranean. They do a great deal of difficult work; they climb bunches of stairs, and they walk... a ton. They stroll, in any event, some portion of separation, to their work environment day by day. They stroll to the rancher's market, the bread kitchen, or the dairy search for a new Greek yogurt. They stroll to their companions' homes, and when they need to accomplish something restful, they go out for a walk. My father sold his vehicle a couple of years prior; he didn't require one in any case.

Presently, on the off chance that you are one of the little levels of individuals who keep a functioning rec center participation, kindly don't stop. Welcoming normal development, a moderate exercise like an everyday walk is a compelling and feasible healthy propensity. I do yoga and CrossFit classes, however, never ordinary. I can all the more effectively fit in a 30-minute walk.

Giggle Often

Are you acquainted with the maxim, "chuckling is the best prescription?" That has positively demonstrated valid on account of the Mediterranean individuals. I can't state this is a trait surprisingly of Mediterranean legacy, yet it is unquestionably obvious in the numerous I know. They are individuals of enormous character. They love to recount stories; their discussions loaded up with humor. There is surely a feeling of need indeed, pay attention to life, yet to do as such with a blissful frame of mind.

Live (More) Simply

Maybe this isn't totally my decision, however individuals of the Mediterranean, or if nothing else the numerous I experienced over the spots I've been—Egypt, Greece, Turkey, and even France—will, in general, have far fewer belongings than I do living here in the States. And I've additionally seen that they settle on stewardship choices with regards to day by day needs. Take food, for instance; Mediterranean people don't purchase a lot of anyone fixing. The whole idea of purchasing in mass stays unfamiliar to them. Eating matters naturally, and they wouldn't fret making different excursions to the market by walking, for the most part. Recipes like fattoush where day-old bread is utilized, or paella where remains are transformed into a dazzling flavor-stuffed rice dish, are two instances of delightful approaches to limiting waste.

Benefits of the Mediterranean Diet

A ton of researchers accepts the Mediterranean Diet is the highest quality level in healthy eating. New investigations show up consistently on driving logical diaries, supporting the restorative effect of the Mediterranean Diet.

These are a few instances of concentrates affirming its medical advantages:

1. Boost your heart wellbeing: Diet alone could help your heart wellbeing.

2. Reach your optimal weight: People following a Mediterranean style diet have all the more long haul benefits and get in shape securely.

3. Control your glucose: Mediterranean diet could assist you with averting high glucose.

4. Improve bones wellbeing: People from the Mediterranean nations have lower paces of hip breaks.

5. Improve your cerebrum wellbeing: Antioxidants found in fruits and vegetables assume a significant job in the psychological limit.

(*) Please note that your outcomes may shift, and you may not get similar outcomes when utilizing this program because of contrasts in your individual history, hereditary qualities, and individual inspiration. Counsel your doctor before starting any sustenance program.

At the point when you consider Mediterranean food, your brain may go-to pizza and pasta from Italy or sheep cleaves from Greece, yet these dishes don't fit into the healthy dietary plans publicized as "Mediterranean." A genuine Mediterranean diet depends on the district's customary fruits, vegetables, beans, nuts, seafood, olive oil, and dairy—with maybe a glass or two of red wine. That is the manner by which the occupants of Crete, Greece, and southern Italy ate around 1960, when their paces of constant disease were among the most reduced on the planet and their future among the most noteworthy, notwithstanding having just constrained restorative administrations.

And the genuine Mediterranean diet is about something other than eating crisp, wholesome food. Every day physical action and offering suppers to others are essential components of the Mediterranean Diet Pyramid. Together, they can profoundly affect your temperament and emotional well-being and assist you with encouraging profound gratefulness for the delights of eating healthy and heavenly foods.

Obviously, making changes to your diet is once in a while easy, particularly in case you're attempting to move away from the accommodation of prepared and takeout foods. Be that as it may, the Mediterranean diet can be cheap just as a wonderful and extremely healthy approach to eating. Changing from pepperoni and pasta to fish and avocados may require some exertion. However, you could before long be on the way to a more beneficial and longer life.

Medical advantages of a Mediterranean diet

A conventional Mediterranean diet comprising of huge amounts of new fruits and vegetables, nuts, fish and olive oil—combined with physical movement—can diminish your danger of genuine mental and physical medical issues by:

Averting coronary illness and strokes. Following a Mediterranean diet restricts your admission of refined pieces of bread, prepared foods, and red meat, and energizes drinking red wine rather than hard alcohol—all factors that can help counteract coronary illness and stroke.

They are keeping you coordinated. In case you're a more established grown-up, the supplements picked up with a Mediterranean diet may lessen your danger of creating muscle shortcoming and different indications of delicacy by around 70 percent.

You are lessening the danger of Alzheimer's. Research recommends that the Mediterranean diet may improve cholesterol, glucose levels, and generally speaking vein wellbeing, which thusly may diminish your danger of Alzheimer's disease or dementia.

Dividing the danger of Parkinson's disease: The significant levels of cancer prevention agents in the Mediterranean diet can keep cells from experiencing a harming procedure called oxidative pressure, in this manner cutting the danger of Parkinson's disease down the middle.

Expanding life span: By diminishing your danger of creating coronary illness or malignant growth with the Mediterranean diet, you're lessening your danger of death at any age by 20%.

Securing against type 2 diabetes: A Mediterranean diet is wealthy in fiber, which processes gradually, prevents enormous swings in glucose, and can assist you with keeping up a healthy weight.

Myths and facts about the Mediterranean diet

Following a Mediterranean diet has numerous benefits. However, there are still a ton of misguided judgments on precisely how to exploit the lifestyle to lead a more beneficial, longer life. Coming up next are a few myths and facts about the Mediterranean diet.

Myths and facts of a Mediterranean diet

Myth 1: It costs a ton to eat along these lines.

Fact: If you're creating dinners out of beans or lentils as your principle wellspring of protein and staying with generally plants and whole grains, at that point, the Mediterranean diet is more affordable than serving dishes of bundled or prepareald foods.

Myth 2: One glass of wine is useful for your heart, at that point, three glasses is multiple times as healthy.

Fact: Moderate measures of red wine (one beverage daily for women; two for men) unquestionably has special medical advantages for your heart, yet drinking a lot of has the contrary impact. Anything over two glasses of wine can really be terrible for your heart.

Myth 3: Eating huge dishes of pasta and bread is the Mediterranean way.

Fact: Typically, Mediterraneans don't eat a colossal plate of pasta the manner in which Americans do. Rather, pasta is normally a side dish with around a 1/2-cup to 1-cup serving size. The remainder of their plate comprises of salads, vegetables, fish or a little segment of natural, grass-encouraged meat, and maybe one cut of bread.

Myth 4: The Mediterranean diet is just about the food.

Fact: The food is a colossal piece of the diet; truly, however, don't disregard different ways the Mediterranean's live their lives. At the point when they plunk down for supper, they don't sit before a TV or eat in a surge; they plunk down for a casual, relaxed feast with others, which might be similarly as significant for your wellbeing as what is on your plate. Mediterranean's additionally appreciate a lot of physical activity.

Step by step instructions to roll out the improvement

In case you're feeling overwhelmed by the idea of changing your eating propensities to a Mediterranean diet, here are a few proposals to kick you off:

Eat loads of vegetables. Attempt a basic plate of cut tomatoes sprinkled with olive oil and disintegrated feta cheddar, or burden your dainty outside layer pizza with peppers and mushrooms rather than hotdog and pepperoni. Salads, soups, and crudité platters are likewise incredible approaches to stack up on vegetables.

Continuously have breakfast. Natural products, whole grains, and other fiber-rich foods are an incredible method to begin your day, keeping you agreeably full for a considerable length of time.

Eat seafood two times every week. Fish, for example, fish, salmon, herring, sablefish (dark cod), and sardines are wealthy in Omega-3 unsaturated fats, and shellfish like mussels, clams, and mollusks have comparable benefits for mind and heart wellbeing.

Cook a veggie-lover feast one night seven days. On the off chance that it's useful, you can hop on the "Meatless Mondays" pattern of previous meat on the primary day of the week, or basically pick a day where you fabricate suppers around beans, whole grains, and vegetables. When you get its hang, attempt two evenings per week.

Appreciate dairy items with some restraint. The USDA prescribes constraining soaked fat to close to 10% of your day by day calories (around 200 calories for the vast majority). That still enables you to appreciate dairy items, for example, regular (natural) cheddar, Greek or plain yogurt.

For dessert, eat the crisp natural product. Rather than a dessert, cake, or other heated merchandise, decide on strawberries, crisp figs, grapes, or apples.

Utilize great fats. Extra-virgin olive oil, nuts, sunflower seeds, olives, and avocados are extraordinary wellsprings of healthy fats for your day by day suppers.

What to do about mercury in fish

Regardless of all the medical advantages of seafood, about all fish and shellfish contain hints of contaminations, including the lethal metal mercury.

These rules can assist you with settling on the most secure decisions.

- ❖ The centralization of mercury and different contaminations increments in bigger fish, so it's ideal to abstain from eating huge fish like shark, swordfish, tilefish, and ruler mackerel.

- ❖ Most grown-ups can securely eat around 12 ounces (two 6-ounce servings) of different sorts of cooked seafood seven days.

- ❖ Pay consideration regarding nearby seafood warnings to learn if fish you've gotten is sheltered to eat.

- ❖ For women who are pregnant, nursing moms, and youngsters matured 12 and more youthful, pick fish and shellfish that are 1 in mercury, for example, shrimp, canned light fish, salmon, Pollock, or catfish. Due to its higher mercury content, eat close to 6 ounces (one normal feast) of tuna fish every week.

Make eating times a social encounter

The straightforward demonstration of conversing with a companion or cherished over the supper table can assume a major job in mitigating pressure and boosting state of mind. Eating with others can likewise anticipate overeating, making it as healthy for your waistline for what it's worth for your viewpoint. Switch off the TV and PC, set away your cell phone, and interface with somebody over a supper.

Assemble the family and keep awake to date with one another's every day lives. Standard family suppers give solace to kids and are an incredible method to screen their eating propensities too.

Offer suppers with others to expand your informal community. On the off chance that you live alone, cook some extra and welcome a companion, collaborator, or neighbor to go along with you.

Cook with others. Welcome a companion to share shopping and cooking duties regarding a

Mediterranean feast. Cooking with others can be a fun method to develop connections, and parting the expenses can make it less expensive for both of you.

Speedy beginning to a Mediterranean diet

The simplest method to roll out the improvement to a Mediterranean diet is, to begin with, little steps. You can do this by:

- ❖ Sautéing food in olive oil rather than margarine.
- ❖ Eating more fruits and vegetables by getting a charge out of salad as a starter or side dish, eating on a natural product, and adding veggies to different dishes.
- ❖ Choosing whole grains rather than refined pieces of bread, rice, and pasta.
- ❖ Substituting fish for red meat, at any rate, two times seven days.
- ❖ Limit high-fat dairy by changing to skim or 1% milk from 2% or whole milk

Rather than this: Try this Mediterranean choice:

Chips, pretzels, saltines and farm dip Carrots, celery, broccoli, and salsa

White rice with pan-seared meat Quinoa with pan-seared vegetables

Sandwiches with white bread or rolls Sandwich fillings in whole-wheat tortillas

Icecream Pudding made with skim or 1% milk

The benefits of the Mediterranean Diet Juice

We, as a whole, realize that fruits and vegetables are an essential piece of the Mediterranean Diet, and they ought to be devoured every day. One method for devouring fruits is by drinking their organic product juice. Mediterranean diet juices can and ought to be devoured day by day, and they fall in the Mediterranean diet drinks classification that we have talked about in one of our past articles.

The benefits from the utilization, drinking, of juices, are numerous, and it depends fundamentally on the sort of juice we drink and the sort of need our body has. Juices "cover-up" in them healthful parts that are required by our body for its smooth and ordinary activity. The Mediterranean organic product juices are viewed as the dietary partner of our body since the benefits coming about because of the juices are numerous and multidimensional!

Fruits and their juices invigorate the body and give it the additional vitality required for the day by day exercises, because of the fact that they contain common sugars, also called starches. Juices give the truly necessary, hydration to the body since water is their significant constituent. Despite the fact that juices ought to be devoured as crisp as could be expected under the circumstances, it is significant that non-concentrated juices are additionally helpful to our body since they don't experience any sort of handling and water and sugar are neither evacuated nor included, consequently keeping the juice as near their unique state as could be allowed. Fruits like the ones having a place with the berry family, similar to raspberry, blueberry and strawberry, pomegranate, and the citrus fruits have expanded cancer prevention agent properties; they contain Vitamin A, B, E and polyphenols, properties which invigorate our body and make us more grounded.

We will give a short rundown of Mediterranea diet juices, which we accept is the most widely recognized as well as the ones who will carry the most healthful advantage to your body. Mediterranean diet juices are only a subset of the general gathering of the Mediterranean Drinks displayed in a past article.

Squeezed orange: Orange juice, OJ, contains Vitamin C, which sustains the bodyguard, adds to the vitality change inside the body while simultaneously improves the assimilation of iron by the body and to the strength of the skin. OJ contains magnesium, and a follow component which is significant for the bone wellbeing. The folic corrosive, which can be found in the Orange Juice, serves to the improvement of the vascular framework coming about to the decrease of cardiovascular and mind episodes. Most recent research about Orange juice has demonstrated that it lessens the terrible cholesterol levels.

Pomegranate Juice: Pomegranate juice is wealthy in cancer prevention agents, gives clean insurance to our body, and it hinders the maturing of the phones. It likewise helps in the decrease of the awful cholesterol level while simultaneously it expands the degrees of the great cholesterol. A blended juice of pomegranate in with raspberry juice gives the body a lot of cancer prevention agents.

Mango Juice: It is another juice that is wealthy in cancer prevention agents that help the battle against the maturing of the phones and gives us healthy and glossy skin. Utilization of a mango juice battles the free radicals, which cause the wrinkles all over, while the carotene b, which it contains adds to the soundness of the eyes and the lungs!

Pear Juice: Pears are fruits which can be utilized in salads, Pear Salad with Walnuts and Feta cheddar, they can be effectively devoured every day, and their juice is the perfect juice for a healthy living. This particular juice is a supernatural occurrence juice all alone, yet it tends to be joined with different juices to make them more delectable and more advantageous. Pear juice isn't just plentiful in Calcium and Vitamin C however it additionally contains elevated levels of Potassium, Magnesium, and Phosphorous which are vital components for our body

Grape Juice: The purple shade of the grape juice is particularly significant for the insurance of the synapses. You can improve your memory with the utilization of a glass of grape juice on a successive premise. Grape juice is additionally wealthy in cell reinforcements, which empower the body to battle emotionally any sort of disease.

Beet Juice! Have you at any point an alcoholic glass of beet juice! It's anything but a well-known juice in the western world, and this sort of juice is most likely perhaps the most advantageous juice you will ever have. It causes your body to battle malignant growth as well as serves to your weight loss, on the off chance that you are in that stage. Beet juice helps in the development and advancement of the red platelets. This particular juice is plentiful in Potassium, Iron, Vitamin C, and Magnesium. It likewise helps patients who experience the ill effects of memory loss to recoup and accomplish the most prominent consideration and focus levels. Beet juice is especially significant for the decrease in the effect caused because of menopause.

Grapefruit Juice: it is the perfect juice for a rich breakfast, and this is the explanation it is energetically suggested by an incredible number of Dietitians, in order to accomplish a decent diet and a healthy method for living, similar to the Mediterranean diet. It contains Vitamins, citrus extract, fundamental oils, flavonoids, and lycopene, which have serious cancer prevention agent activity.

Squeezed apple: Most ongoing examinations have demonstrated that the squeezed apple, which isn't clear it is more beneficial than the reasonable squeezed apple due to the polyphenols that it contains. It is a juice plentiful in Vitamin C and different components that help in the creation of a solid bone structure. It contains cancer prevention agents, something which revives the body without forcing any fats.

Pineapple juice: It is a juice with the light and extraordinary taste and fragrance offering a special tasting experience giving every one of us the healthful segments of the pineapple. The unique compound bromelain that it is found on the pineapple juice has the property to break proteins and help the absorption procedure. Pineapple juice is plentiful in nutrient C.

Tomato juice: This is a decent chance to get out in our psyches that tomato is anything but a vegetable, yet it is a natural product! It is a natural product wealthy in lycopene, a component that gives it the red shading and decreases the danger of malignant growth, particularly prostate disease. Tomato juice has not many calories; however, it is plentiful in Vitamin C. One glass of tomato juice contains half of our every day needs in Vitamin C.

Peach juice: Peach juice is a decent wellspring of solvent fiber in this way, contributing to the decrease of the LDL cholesterol. It has a couple of calories and an incredible number of nutrients. Because of the gathering of nutrients, it has, particularly Vitamins C and E, it shields our body from the gastrointestinal issue, and it is particularly prescribed for the smooth activity of the colon. The utilization of peach juice helps in the unwinding of the body and aids in the concealment of the menopause syndromes.

Morello, Black cherry, Juice: This is another sort of juice you can't discover effectively; however, in certain Mediterranean nations like Greece and Turkey, this sort of juice is outstanding. It has a specific and unmistakable taste and fragrance, and this is the explanation it is utilized in numerous pharmaceutical arrangements and syrups. It is an uncommon sort of cherry which was utilized widely during the medieval occasions for therapeutic purposes. Each glass of this sort of juice offers to the body starches which revive the body and give us vitality!

Juices are a significant and nourishing enhancement of our ordinary diet, and it is dependent upon us to choose the sort of juice we will have depending on the time, in the event that it will go with our feast or on the off chance that it will be taken previously or after an activity. Mediterranean diet advances the utilization of new juices of any sort, and juices are a piece of the "every day utilization" step of the Mediterranean diet pyramid. Simply pursue your heart and want for the juice you will have, and you will appreciate the wholesome benefits minutes after the fact.

Foods to Eat

This is an example food list:

New organic product. Have 3 or 4 bits of natural product consistently. Make one of these fruits an orange; they are high in cancer prevention agents and phytochemicals, substances that secure us against issues. Berries, (for example, strawberries, blueberries, raspberries) are likewise an unquestionable requirement in this diet due to their cancer prevention agents. In the event that you need to pursue a Mediterranean diet, eat some organic products for dessert. That is the means by which Mediterraneans eat their natural product a large portion of the occasions.

Veggies. Have a salad in your principle dinners. Utilize olive oil and lemon for dressing; This is an incredible cancer prevention agent mix. Tomatoes and tomato items are a staple food in the Mediterranean diet; they contain lycopene. Cut a whole tomato and spread it with olive oil and some basil as a major aspect of your side dish or remember them for eyour salads. Zucchini is additionally an awesome supplement; sauté them with olive oil.

Whole Grains: Have a bit of whole wheat or whole grain bread with your fundamental dinners (aside from with pasta). Have whole wheat pasta 2 or 3 times each week. It is low in calories, and the fiber upgrades the sentiment of totality.

Legumes: Eat dried beans, lentils, or garbanzo beans 2 or 3 times each week. Sustenance specialists at the

Michigan State University disclose to us that eating 2 to 4 cups of cooked legumes consistently could support our heart wellbeing. Dry beans have fiber that could decrease cholesterol from the body. Eat legumes and a bit of whole grain bread to have the ideal protein. Vegetable protein doesn't put a heap on kidneys as creature protein does.

Nuts. Have a handful of nuts as a nibble in your morning break. Nuts are likewise a staple food in Mediterranean nations and are high in monounsaturated fat, the one that doesn't stall out in the corridors. Peruse the food mark and know about parts since nuts are high in calories. Logical examinations have discovered that almonds and walnuts could be the most beneficial decisions.

Olive oil: Utilize olive oil in your suppers both to cook and as a fixing in your salads. Olive oil is the principle wellspring of fat in Mediterranean nations and could be the "cause" of the low frequency of heart issues in those nations [7]. Utilize olive oil and lemon as a plunge in your salads.

Fish and seafood; Have fish and seafood a few times each week. Salmon and sardines are magnificent decisions since they give omega-3 oils, oils that the body needs; however, they can't take in enough amounts.

Garlic and sweet-smelling herbs: Use garlic and sweet-smelling herbs as a sauce. Garlic could be the main supporter of the low occurrence of hypertension in Mediterranean nations [8].

Test Mediterranean Diet Menu

A multi-day diet plan would present changes step by step. Studies have demonstrated that little changes after some time are a successful method to make long-lasting propensities. Start with the end of handled foods and increment products of the soil. Proceed by including more beans and change from different oils (or margarine) to additional virgin olive oil. Farthest point seafood, poultry, and eggs to a couple of times each week each and lessen red meat to close to a bit a month. And at last, spotlight on dairy items and maintain a strategic distance from milk, cream, and margarine.

It is hard to pick only one menu. However, this is what daily of suppers may resemble:

➢ Breakfast: Greek yogurt beat with berries and walnuts; Coffee or tea

➢ Lunch: Lentil soup with wash chard beat with tzatziki sauce; Hummus and pita

➢ Snack: Whole grain saltines and cheddar

➢ Dinner: Roasted cod matched with a wheat berry salad comprising of olive oil vinaigrette, feta, parsley, and tomatoes and a glass of red wine

➢ Dessert: Fresh organic product showered with nectar

How to Lose Weight While on the Mediterranean Diet?

sserEat at least five servings of fruits and vegetables every day. Pick foods plentiful in fiber, nutrients, and phytonutrients. Eat legumes, in any event, eight times each week. Legumes are low fat, fiber-filled, and a decent wellspring of protein. Point of confinement refined grains and pick whole grains. Lower fat dairy choices ought to supplant full-fat dairy items. Olive oil would be restricted to a tablespoon every day. The human body requires dietary fat, and plant-based olive oil is a heart-healthy decision.

Fish, eggs, and poultry ought to be restricted to close to two servings each, every week. These are great wellsprings of protein. However, they contain a bigger number of calories than legumes. Wine ought to be constrained to one glass for each day. A four-ounce glass of red wine is brimming with cancer prevention agents; however, it contains 100 to 120 calories.

Eat organic products for dessert. Expend close to 2 eggs per week. Supplant spread with olive oil for cooking. Utilize nectar to improve (no sugar). Eat red meats once per month. Put in 30 min. of moderate physical activity every day.

Step by step instructions to Follow The Mediterranean Diet: Advice for Beginners

In case you're brand new to eating the Mediterranean way, "start with basic swaps."

– The main week, get some quality additional virgin olive oil and start utilizing olive oil as your essential cooking oil (instead of spread, fat, or different oils).

– The following week, attempt to join 1 or 2 seafood-based suppers, and/or 1 or 2 meatless dinners. Load up on healthy tidbits and things like hummus and veggies, just as a crisp or dried organic product.

– To end your suppers, instead of treats, appreciate a little bit of generally created cheddar like feta, Parmigiano-

Reggiano or Pecorino Romano with a handful of dried apricots, figs, or fruits.

THE DIFFERENT WAYS TO PURSUE THE MEDITERRANEAN DIET (RECIPES INCLUDED)

1-Eliminate quick foods. For huge numbers of us living in America, this is one of the harder changes and may take some time. To begin with, take a stab at swapping a cheap food feast with a custom made one. For instance, if it's chicken wings you ache for, make them Greek-style like in this formula! Or on the other hand, if it's sweet potato fries (my own extravagance), take a stab at heating them in olive oil with a sprinkle of Mediterranean flavors like in this formula.

The fact of the matter is, locate a more advantageous custom made option in contrast to your preferred quick foods.

2-Eat more vegetables, fruits, grains, and legumes. The base of the Mediterranean diet pyramid should make up the base of each dinner. At the point when you can, settle on vegan courses like this Cauliflower and Chickpea Stew or Spicy Spinach and Lentil Soup. Depend more on fulfilling season pressed salads to make up a decent segment of your plate — a few thoughts: Kidney Bean Salad; Mediterranean Chickpea Salad; Greek Salad; Balela Salad.

3-Swap fats. A decent spot to begin is by supplanting spread with olive oil in your cooking.

4-Reduce your admission of greasy red meats… a great deal. Eat progressively lean proteins–fish around two times each week; and poultry with some restraint. A couple of top picks are this Easy Baked Salmon; Shrimp Skewers; One-Pan Halibut and Vegetables; Mediterranean Grilled Chicken; and Egg Shakshuka!

You can positively still eat red meat once in a while (constrained); however, pick less fatty cuts. Sheep is frequently the red meat of decisions in Greece and other Mediterranean nations. You may get a kick out of the chance to attempt: Kofta Kebobs, Grilled Lamb Chops with Mint Quinoa, or Moussaka (Greek eggplant and sheep goulash). For unique events, I enthusiastically suggest Leg of Lamb with Potatoes.

5-Eat some dairy and eggs. Utilization of dairy items (with some restraint) gives medical advantages, including the lower danger of diabetes, metabolic syndrome, cardiovascular disease, and corpulence. Tragically, as per USDA, in excess of 80 percent of the whole U.S. populace doesn't meet the day by day dairy admission recommendation! We are not looking at fixing everything with heaps of handled cheddar. In any case, maybe for a tidbit, swap your chips for low-fat Greek yogurt. Include a sprinkle of feta cheddar to your salad, or swap mayonnaise or your sandwich spread for low-fat Tzatziki sauce.

6-You've heard this before, "don't drink your calories." In the Mediterranean diet, this means drinking more water and swapping calorie-loaded Margaritas for an infrequent glass of red wine.

7-Share, however, many suppers with others as would be prudent. These aides in a few different ways. Investing energy with friends and family diminishes pressure and hoists our states of mind. In any case, being intentional, and backing off to associate with others, likewise enables us to control our bits.

Step by Step Guide to Eating Mediterranean

It is really evident that the Mediterranean Diet is probably the most advantageous approach to eat on the planet. There are presently thousands of concentrates that demonstrate that changing to this well-known method for eating can diminish your danger of coronary illness, disease, diabetes, corpulence, and even dementia, asthma, and Alzheimer's. The issue is that there is disarray about what a Mediterranean diet truly is. In the event that we go to a café and request Mediterranean chicken pasta that accompanies a half-pound of spaghetti, another half pound (or a greater amount of) chicken, a half-pound of cheddar, and just a scarcely recognizable measure of vegetables than that is certifiably not a conventional Mediterranean dish!

The foods of the Mediterranean are very differed. A regular Turkish feast is unique in relation to a customary Spanish or Egyptian one, yet what isn't diverse are the base fixings. Olive oil, vegetables, organic product, beans, nuts, seeds with certain grains, creature items, and moderate measures of liquor (few out of every odd nation) are the staples of the diet. The base diet of these nations is heart-healthy, mitigating, and for the most part, exceptionally "bravo" foods. They are foods such are reality continuing rather than life exhausting. The individuals of the Mediterranean praise cooking, eating, and mingling. They don't go on diets or tally their calories; they simply appreciate.

Changing to any better approach for eating can feel overpowering, making individuals bound to surrender, which is the reason we are recommending you pursue our "slowly and carefully" approach. Rather than attempting to "become" Mediterranean medium-term, we suggest facilitating in overtime of half a month or even months. Huge numbers of you are deciding to take a stab at eating the Mediterranean due to wellbeing reasons, yet we figure you will remain in view of the lifestyle and the delectable food.

The Differences Between Mediterranean Diet Cuisines

A Greek Mediterranean diet plan (or a Cretan Diet) is a heart-healthy plan dependent on foods that are generally eaten in Greece, Crete, and Southern Italy.

The greater part of these food varieties shares similar standards. Plant-based foods make up most of the diet, with the principle fat source originating from olive oil. Devouring fish and seafood week after week. Wine with some restraint. Red meat every so often, when a month. Starches as whole grains. New fruits and vegetables. The essential protein source originates from low-fat sources like beans and seafood. One-half cup of beans has about a similar protein content as an ounce of meat with no immersed fat. Eggs, poultry, and seafood in a restricted sum every week.

Who Invented the Mediterranean Diet

The history of the Mediterranean diet has millenarian starting points. Its standards were at that point being used from the fourth century under the Roman domain. The diet pulled in global enthusiasm after an examination led by Dr. Ancel keys toward the finish of the Second universal war. Dr. Keys saw how the populace in the Cilento (southern Italy), had a more

[64]

prominent life span, minor frequency of heart issues. The Doctor comprehended that it was because of the nutritious routine they pursued. At that point, he chose to attempt an "Investigation of the seven nations" [6] so as to check the wellbeing similitudes of various Mediterranean populaces. Ancel Keys lived in a little town of anglers (Poplars) in the basics of Pollica in the area of Salerno, Italy, for a long time. He died in November 2004 at 100 years age.

The Mediterranean diet has its beginnings in a segment of land thought about one of a kind in its sort, the Mediterranean bowl, which students of history called "the support of society," in light of the fact that inside its geological fringes the whole history of the old world occurred.

At its banks extended the valley of the Nile, the site of an old and propelled human advancement, and the two extraordinary bowls of the Tigris and Euphrates, which were the earth of the development of the

Sumerians, Assyrians, Babylonians, and Persians. In the Mediterranean locale emerged the intensity of the Cretans. At that point rose the Phoenicians and the scholarly Greeks up to the developing intensity of Rome, which enabled the region to turn into the "great land" between the East and the West. From that time, the Mediterranean turned into the gathering spot of individuals who, with their contacts, have every now and then adjusted culture, customs, dialects, religions, and perspectives about changing and changing lifestyles with the advancement of history. The conflict of these two cultures delivered their halfway joining, so even the eating propensities converged to some extent.

The starting points of the "Mediterranean Diet" are lost in time since they sink into the eating propensities for the Middle Ages, in which the old Roman custom - on the model of the Greek - recognized in bread, wine and oil items and image of rustic culture and rural (and images chose of the new confidence), enhanced by sheep cheddar, vegetables (leeks, mallow, lettuce, chicory, mushrooms), little meat and a solid inclination for fish and seafood (of which antiquated Rome was exceptionally avaricious). The rich classes adored the crisp fish (who ate generally seared in olive oil or flame-broiled) and seafood, particularly clams, eating crude or singed. Captives of Rome, nonetheless, was ordained poor food comprises of bread and a large portion of a pound of olives and olive oil a month, with some salted fish, once in a while a little meat. The Roman convention before long conflicted with the style of food imported from the culture of the Germanic people groups, for the most part, travelers, and living in close congruity with the woodland, got from the equivalent, with chasing, cultivating and assembling, a large portion of the food assets. Raised pigs of fat, generally utilized in the kitchen, and developed vegetables in little gardens near the camps. A couple of grains developed were not used to make bread, however lager. The conflict of these two cultures delivered their fractional joining, so even the eating propensities converged to a limited extent. Notwithstanding, the Roman culture showed itself reluctant to change the style of "The Mediterranean" of bolstering with that primitive. The major part of the Mediterranean diet, which is the group of three oil bread and wine, were sent out rather in areas of mainland Europe by the ascetic requests, which moved in those locales to proselytize those people groups. Bread, oil, and wine were, in fact, the focal components of the Christian ceremony, yet they have later embraced additionally in the sustaining of the everyday citizens of Europe. The new food culture conceived from the association and the combination between dietary examples of two distinct human advancements, the Christian Roman Empire and the Germanic, crossed with the progression of time with a third convention or that of the Arab world, which had built up its own special food culture on the southern shores of the Mediterranean.

Just Muslims gave a lift to a reestablishment of agriculture that affected the food model with the presentation of plant species known or utilized distinctly by the wealthier social classes, due to the significant expenses, for example, sugar stick, rice, citrus, eggplant, spinach, and flavors, just as discovered use in the cooking of southern Europe, rose water, oranges, lemons, almonds, and pomegranates.

Islamic culture, in this manner, takes an interest in the change and change of the social solidarity of the Mediterranean, which Rome had constructed, and gives a conclusive commitment to the new culinary model that was framing. A critical number of foods, passed by Muslims on Latin, drag their planning strategies and recipes.

Another occasion of extraordinary recorded effect was, as it is outstanding, the disclosure of America by

Europeans. This revelation is likewise reflected in a "buy" with respect to the culinary custom of new foodstuffs, for example, potatoes, tomatoes, corn, peppers, and stew, just as various assortments of beans. The tomato, "extraordinary interest," fancy organic product just belatedly thought to be consumable, was the main red vegetable that advanced our bushel of plants and later turned into an image of the Mediterranean cooking.

In the event that the centrality of vegetables is one of the most unique characters of the Mediterranean convention, it is critical to recollect the job of grains as the premise of basic cooking and as a weapon of day by day endurance, as a result of their "capacity to fill" decreasing cravings for food of poor classes. The kind of oats devoured, just as the methods of change, accept various features relying upon the topographical undertones and conventions that describe the populaces of the nations verging on the

Mediterranean. Bread, polenta, couscous, soups, paella, and pasta are various approaches to devour grains.

This recorded way simply depicted permits recognizing numerous similitudes between the Mediterranean diet and current diet of our progenitors to exhibit the nearness of a genuine way that from the sustaining of the Egyptians to the disclosure of America prompted the presentation of new foods, giving us the Mediterranean diet as we probably are aware today.

The Mediterranean Diet is a nourishing model, so all around valued that has a place with the social, verifiable, social, regional, and ecological and is firmly identified with the lifestyle of the Mediterranean people groups since their commencement. The Candidature Dossier submitted to UNESCO characterizes the Mediterranean Diet as follows:"... getting from the Greek word "diaita"- lifestyle,

lifestyle - it is a social practice dependent on all the "savoir-faire," information, customs going from the landscape to the table and covering the Mediterranean Basin, cultures, collecting, angling, preservation, handling, arrangement, cooking and specifically the manner in which we expend, i.e., sociability."

The Mediterranean diet, referred to basically as a food model, improves the quality and wellbeing of foods and their connection to the land of birthplace. It offers basic cooking, yet wealthy in the creative mind and tastes, exploiting all parts of a healthy diet. It is a moral decision that jams the conventions and customs of the people groups of the Mediterranean Basin. Nourishing can significantly influence the wellbeing of people; this is on the grounds that a decent dietary status keeps up a decent degree of wellbeing and counteractive action of metabolic diseases, for example, weight, diabetes, hypertension, and so on. The Mediterranean Diet is additionally an "asset for reasonable improvement is significant for every one of the nations verging on the Mediterranean, to the financial and cultural impact the food covers all through the district and the capacity to motivate a feeling of progression and character for nearby individuals."

Mediterranean diet: eating practices and lifestyles

The revelation of the medical advantages of the Mediterranean Diet is credited to the American researcher Ancel Keys of the University of Minnesota School of Power, which called attention to the relationship between's cardiovascular disease and diet just because. Ancel Keys, in the fifties, was struck by a marvel, which proved unable, from the outset, give a full explanation. The poor populace of communities of southern Italy was, against all forecasts, a lot more advantageous than the rich residents of New York, both of their own family members who emigrated in before decades in the United States. Keys recommended this relied upon food and attempted to approve his unique knowledge, concentrating on foods that made up the diet of these populaces. In this manner, he drove the renowned "Seven Countries Study" (directed in Finland, Holland, Italy, United States, Greece, Japan, and Yugoslavia), so as to record the connection between lifestyles, sustenance and cardiovascular disease between various populaces, including through cross-sectional examinations, having the option to demonstrate deductively the dietary benefit of the Mediterranean diet and its commitment to the strength of the populace that embraced it.

From this investigation rose plainly, as the populaces that had received a diet-dependent on the Mediterranean Diet exhibited a low pace of cholesterol in the blood and, therefore, a base level of coronary illness. This was for the most part because of the ample utilization of olive oil, bread, pasta, vegetables, herbs, garlic, red onions, and different foods of vegetable inception contrasted with a fairly moderate utilization of meat.

The American nutritionist portrayed the Mediterranean diet along these lines: "... natively constructed minestrone, pasta everything being equal, with tomato sauce and a sprinkling of Parmesan, just at times enhanced with a couple of bits of meat or presented with a little fish of the spot beans and macaroni ..., so much bread, never expelled from the stove in excess of a couple of hours before being eaten, and nothing with which spread it, heaps of crisp vegetables sprinkled with olive oil, a little part of meat or fish perhaps two or three times each week and in every case new organic product for dessert".

Beginning from Keys' investigations, numerous other logical researchers have broken down the relationship between dietary propensities and ceaseless diseases. It is currently conceivable to state that there is an intermingling of evaluations concurred toward full acknowledgment of the helpful characteristics of the Mediterranean method for eating. Numerous examinations and clinical preliminaries have demonstrated that the Mediterranean diet diminishes the danger of cardiovascular disease and metabolic syndrome. Specifically has been placed into proof an astounding abatement of stomach circuit, an expansion in high thickness lipoprotein (HDL), a diminishing in triglycerides, a bringing down of circulatory strain, and a lessening in the convergence of glucose in the blood.

Nonetheless, we should bring up that the Mediterranean diet can't create, without anyone else's input, the benefits recorded above on the off chance that you don't change simultaneously other hazard factors (clearly those modifiable). In fact, ischemic coronary illness depends not just on blunders in the creation of the diet, to which joins a prevailing job, yet in addition by different factors, for example, a decreased or missing physical action, caloric admission in abundance of the vitality needs of the living being, the nearness of metabolic diseases, for example, diabetes and stoutness, stress, cigarette smoking, elevated levels of homocysteine in the blood, significant levels of triglycerides. In this way, it isn't astounding that about a portion of all instances of stroke happens in people with an ordinary degree of cholesterol in the blood. To anticipate a respiratory failure is in this manner basic to take not just a reasonable diet (as is without a doubt the Mediterranean diet) yet, in addition, a healthy lifestyle (as Ancel Keys had just called attention to).

In 2007, an examination directed by the National Institutes of Health indicated that moderate physical movement is related to a diminishing in mortality from cardiovascular disease.

In fact, physical movement decreases some hazard factors for cardiovascular disease, for example, hypertension, insulin opposition, hypertriglyceridemia, low HDL, and the nearness of stoutness. Additionally, practice, coupled with legitimate nourishment, can diminish the blood levels of LDL. Different benefits incorporate the beginning of atherosclerosis, since practice improves myocardial capacity, expands the vasodilator limit, muscle tone, and diminishes incendiary pressure.

You may ask why you have spent such huge numbers of words, for a long time or somewhere in the vicinity, to upgrade a diet that needn't bother with any presentation. The explanation is that the pattern away from the conventional diet for food designs commonplace of the wealthy society has been continuous for a long time. The Mediterranean Diet is along these lines described by the fair utilization of foods wealthy in fiber, cancer prevention agents, and unsaturated fats, a healthy methodology intended to lessen the utilization of creature fats and cholesterol in a diet with a fitting harmony between vitality admission and use. The connections between the macronutrient vitality answer to those perceived as sufficient, ie, 55–60% of sugars of which 80% complex starches (bread, pasta, rice), 10–15% of proteins about 60% of creature starting point (particularly white meat, fish), 25–30% fat (for the most part olive oil). The rules created by nutritionists to improve the eating propensities for shoppers can be spoken to by a powerful picture, the "Food Pyramid" The U.S. Branch of Agriculture, which basically speaks to a reasonable and adjusted method for eating, showing the extents and the frequencies with which foods ought to be expended, style that harmonizes with the Mediterranean Model recognized by the physiologist Ancel Keys.

The Mediterranean diet food pyramid

The primary ideas of the Food Pyramid are the "proportionality," that is the perfect measure of foods to look over for each gathering, the "partition" standard amount of food in grams, which is accepted as the unit of estimation to be a reasonable encouraging, the "assortment," i.e., the significance of changing the decisions inside a food gathering, and "balance" in the utilization of specific foods, for example, fat or desserts. As should be obvious, at the base of the pyramid are grains, trailed by fruits and vegetables, legumes, olive oil, low-fat cheddar, and yogurt, which ought to be eaten day by day. Meat isn't rejected; however, it is given the inclination to that of chicken, hare, and turkey than a hamburger. Alongside fish and eggs ought to be eaten a couple of times each week, for the inventory of excellent protein. Hamburger or red meat ought to be eaten a couple of times each month.

Each gathering incorporates foods, which are significantly "comparable" on the healthful plan, as in they give almost a similar kind of supplements. Clearly, inside a similar gathering, foods in spite of being homogeneous with one another can have little contrasts as far as quality and amount of patrimony in supplements. Be that as it may, this doesn't influence the idea of "compatibility" of foods. The last, in fact, in the event that they have a place with a similar gathering, being healthfully proportionate, might be substituted for one another without, nonetheless, influencing the sufficiency of the diet, gave you go along the assortment. In nature doesn't exist a "total" food; for example, it contains every one of the supplements the body needs, and that is the reason it is important to fluctuate, however much as could be expected food decisions and appropriately consolidate foods from the various gatherings. A differed Diet not just evades the danger of uneven dietary characters and conceivable ensuing metabolic irregular characteristics; however, it likewise fulfills the flavor of battling the repetitiveness of flavors. Each gathering expected is spoken to by in any event a part of the foods that establish it, to change the decisions inside a similar gathering (23). Table 1 shows the Wellness Quantity (WQ) and their weights (the crude and net waste). The idea of sum is utilized to point our consideration on• Portion of food, as amount in grams, which is perfect with the prosperity of our body, so there is nothing more than a bad memory foods or terrible, yet their impact relies upon the sum expended every day, the decision of a fitting number of bits of food should cover all the food bunches in the pyramid day by day to make certain to take every one of the supplements; physical movement, not to fall into an inactive lifestyle, the WQ of reference is a brief stroll at a lively pace, we suggest at any rate 2 WQ/day which is 30 minutes walk likewise distinct during the day. The QB of food and development, if appropriately adjusted to the necessities of the individual, permit arranging the lifestyles towards harmony between food admission and vitality use. Along these lines, you can maintain a strategic distance from the overweight and battling stoutness that inclines the living being to an expanded danger of metabolic diseases (diabetes, hypertension, and so forth), cardiovascular diseases, and even malignant growth.

Grains and tubers

The primary gathering, the oats, and tubers incorporate bread, pasta, rice, corn, oats, grain, spelled, and potatoes. This gathering must be available inconsistently encouraging (ideally with whole foods since more fiber-rich) and in a few bits, in light of the fact that these foods are the most significant wellspring of starch, effectively usable vitality from our body. This doesn't imply that grains ought to be eaten in excessive amounts, however, to be devoured in relation to their needs. It is adequate to state, by method, for instance, 120g of uncooked pasta gives 427 calories, 80g is comparable to 285 calories too, and 55g to 196 calories. In addition, a portion of these foods contain nutrients of the B gathering and a decent lot of protein (as in they come up short on some fundamental amino acids in adequate amounts, among which, especially lysine) that, related with legumes, establish a dinner with a high protein admission and high organic worth, practically identical to meat. This mix happens much of the time in our diet since the grains and their subsidiaries are the essential elements for the planning of numerous dishes. The most popular models are the main dishes from grains and vegetables: these dishes, because of the ability of proteins of the oats to be "reciprocal" to the proteins found in legumes, and giving commonly the amino acids of which are uniquely missing (separately lysine for oats and methionine for legumes), understand an improvement of the nature of the two proteins, which on the whole gets like that of meat proteins (24).

Products of the soil

The gathering of fruits and vegetables additionally incorporates crisp legumes like green beans. They should be carefully seasonal and as new as could be expected under the circumstances: just along these lines, they can grow better their quality and are more delicious in light of the fact that aged to the warmth of the sun.

Vegetables and fruits aged in the nursery, be that as it may, require a more noteworthy stock of pesticides and not exploiting the warmth of the sun, they are less plentiful in nutrients and supplements. Fruits and vegetables are a significant wellspring of fiber, Vitamin A (found fundamentally in tomatoes, peppers, carrots, melon, apricots, and so on), Vitamin C (essentially in tomatoes, strawberries, citrus fruits, kiwi, and so on), different nutrients and numerous minerals, similar to potassium. Likewise, fruits and vegetables contain these minor parts (cell reinforcements and others), which play a significant defensive activity for the body and water that can reach even 95% of the weight (watermelon). Besides, contain any significant amounts of dietary fiber (cellulose, hemicellulose, and gelatin), which in spite of having an inborn healthy benefit, has a job in encouraging the intestinal travel and in directing the degrees of blood cholesterol and glucose More predictable is, rather, the commitment in sugar (sucrose and fructose) produced using organic product. It is fundamental that foods in this gathering are available consistently and bounty in sustenance. The job of foods grown from the ground in the diet is likewise connected to its physiological controller of water balance for their significant stockpile of water. Besides, the substance of potassium salts can neutralize the acids emerging from a nourishing today over and over again, wealthy in creature proteins. At long last, we ought not overlook the job of these foods in the avoidance of stoutness, because of their high substance of fiber and water and low in calories that give (12 calories for zucchini, 16 calories for eggplant, 14Kcal for cucumbers, 12 Kcal for fennel and so on) contrasted with the volume ingested and the high satisfying force (24).

Milk and dairy items

The dairy bunch incorporates milk, yogurt, cheddar, and dairy items. This food bunch gives calcium in an exceptionally bioavailable structure, that is effectively absorbed by the body. In addition, these foods contain high organic quality proteins and a few nutrients (B2 and A). Inside the gathering are favored low-fat milk, dairy items, and low-fat cheddar. The calcium in milk (either be incompletely or totally skimmed) and its subsidiaries is the most critical supplement, with the idiosyncrasy to be better assimilated and utilized by the body. The milk contains more than 1g of calcium per liter, white cheddar, as indicated by the innovation of readiness, contains a few more percents so that in the hard cheeses and season, the amount of calcium can be multiple times higher than that present in milk to approach weight. Notwithstanding calcium, these foods give critical measures of proteins of high natural worth; among this casein is the most spoken to (the part that coagulates when the milk sours and which frames the reason for the arrangement of cheddar) and lactalbumin which together establish 3.5%. The utilization of milk is along these lines the most prompt approach to make the supplements normal for the gathering, yet a similarly substantial option is spoken to by yogurt and cheeses, where they exist instances of narrow lactose mindedness, because of the need or nonappearance of an intestinal protein called "lactase," answerable for the breakdown of lactose in the two mixes galactose and glucose (24).

Meat, fish, and eggs

The meat is viewed as a food vital by ideals of its high protein content (from the fifteenth to 25%) and of high natural worth, ready to make all the amino acids important for protein combination (fundamental amino acids) in ideal sums. It likewise gives B-complex nutrients and follows components, especially iron, zinc, and copper. Notwithstanding, be careful not all foods in this gathering are the equivalent: between the meats is smarter to favor those lean, both cow-like and pork, and white meat and fish and better moderate the utilization of fatter meat and more frankfurters. For eggs in healthy subjects is permitted utilization of egg 2–3 times each week. Foods in this gathering must be available in our diet a couple of times each week, except for red meat, which ought to be eaten a couple of times each month. Any food of creature root having a place with this gathering, regardless of whether crisp, chilled and solidified, gives protein of high natural worth, follow components and nutrients of the B complex, remembering for specific thiamine (nutrient B1), niacin (nutrient PP) and nutrient B12, the last is brought on the whole of foods of creature birthplace. A few foods of this gathering additionally give non-insignificant amounts of different minerals, for example, iodine (in fish) and fat-solvent nutrients (nutrient An and D, contained principally in the liver).

The measure of protein contained in the food bunch is equivalent to 18–20% of the all-out weight, with higher qualities for protected meats (salami), where it might reach up to 37% because of the loss of water subsequent to drying.

Dressing fats

The dressing fats bunch incorporates vegetable fats, for example, olive oil (liked) and those of creature beginning: spread, cream, bacon-fat, and fat. Dressing fats upgrade the flavors and give fundamental unsaturated fats to the retention of fat-solvent nutrients, for the arrangement of the cell layer and of some essential components of the cell. Be that as it may, their utilization, mainly on account of creature fats, must be constrained for two reasons: they give numerous calories and, utilized in abundance, speak to a hazard factor for the beginning of heftiness, cardiovascular diseases, and tumors. There is an unmistakable relationship between's the utilization of soaked unsaturated fats and the beginning of Coronary Heart Disease and is along these lines not prescribed to supplant immersed fats with polyunsaturated. Olive oil is a key component in the Mediterranean diet as it prevents cardiovascular disease. The phenols found in olive oil are to be sure amazing cell reinforcements with calming and hostile to thrombotic, and some monounsaturated unsaturated fats found in olive oil are defensive for cardiovascular disease. Consequently, the olive oil is generally alluded to as "sweeper of corridors."

Ends

One might say that the Mediterranean diet isn't just a gigantic abundance of foods and recipes. Yet, also, a significant purpose of contact among individuals and domain: the people groups of the Mediterranean have consistently found in their land their lives, and are conceived from the dirt the greater part of the results of the diet. The relentless assortment of items in the lands of the Mediterranean need to guarantee, whenever expended in a fitting way, all that our body needs to work. Today sustaining has become a significant perspective in the life of each person. The specialty of eating admirably has gotten a model for general society to pursue, but on the other hand, are expanding non-autochthonous lifestyles, which are in some objective populace a fruitful ground to build the number of adepts of these new ways. In the therapeutic field, the diet has gotten one of the most significant perspectives to be observed at all phases of the life of the subject: the anticipation of numerous diseases to diet treatment that discovers increasingly more acknowledgment among doctors and patients. The achievement of the Mediterranean diet is its organization: a shifted diet portrayed by high utilization of vegetables, fruits, grains, legumes, fish, eggs, alongside a moderate admission of meat, oil, and wine. A diet wealthy in convention and a relationship with one dynamic lifestyle is the model that everybody ought to pursue.

MEDITERRANEAN DIET TIPS

The Mediterranean Diet and the Italian Cuisine

Mediterranean Diet is likely the most beneficial diet, healthy method for living, on the planet, and Italian Cuisine is presumably the most well-known food on the planet. What do the two share in for all intents and purposes? Italian cooking is one of the numerous foods in the Mediterranean area, and it is a piece of the Mediterranean Diet and legacy. You can't be following the Med diet without remembering for your diet some Italian foods and be following the Italian food and preparing or getting a charge out of one of the numerous and extraordinary Italian foods.

Italian Cuisine has been as of late casted a ballot as the most famous food on the planet, and 5 out of the main ten cooking styles of the world are from the

Mediterranean bowl and are a piece of the Mediterranean food. Let us investigate a portion of the qualities and separating factors of the Italian cooking that would empower us to understand the genuine benefits and healthy traits of the Italian food and items.

Nature of Ingredients: The fixings utilized in the Italian foods by the Italian gourmet experts are significant since they characterize the flavor of the particular food. The nature of fixings is so significant in Italian cooking, and this is the explanation that in a large portion of the Italian eateries, these fixings are picked or shopped by the gourmet specialists themselves. Italian food and preparing are so shortsighted, few and great quality fixings are utilized with the goal that you would understand what you are eating! So you have to pick the freshest and the best fixings which will be utilized in your cooking to create a top-notch Italian food and for you to be effective and fulfill your clients or visitors. So discussing explicit fixings, let us talk about Parmigiano cheddar. Parmigiano cheddar is exceptional, and on the off chance that you need to get the genuine flavor in your Italian food, at that point, Parmigiano cheddar is the correct approach. Another must be fixing in Italian food is additional virgin olive oil. There is an incredible number of additional virgin oil brands, and even in Italy, there are numerous additional virgin oil assortments. You have to pick the correct additional virgin oil for the correct formula and food you are planning, one which would match and mix with different fixings. Different produce like vegetables, which are utilized in Italian foods, have to do with seasonality. You would need to utilize the freshest which are in the market since the freshest ones are normally the ones in season and the least expensive of the vegetables you may discover in the market. They are the most reasonable and freshest as well as they are the most delectable ones! When you have chosen the quality fixings, the following significant factor is how you pair these fixings. In Italy and the Italian food, what develops in the territory, locally, works and combines best with different elements of the region, so you have to know a tad about local Italian cooking to assemble and coordinate the correct fixings!

Bona fide Italian Products: If you need to utilize credible Italian produce while cooking your preferred Italian foods or while serving your preferred Italian antipasti, you have to know and understand certain names that you may discover on these items. A portion of these names are:

DOP: Denominazione di OrigineProtetta (Protected Designation of Origin): It is the European Union assignment for the prior Italian DOC, which stands for Denominazione Di OrigineControllata (Controlled Designation of Origin).Both DOP and DOC are legitimate to utilize; however, nowadays, DOC is utilized for the most part for wines. The DOP assignment shows that the item was made in a specific territory for which it is ordinary utilizing conventional techniques. It shields customary foods from substandard impersonations! The law securing DOP items indicates the fixings and creation strategies. It can likewise indicate the race of the creature, the milk or meat originates from, for cheddar and Salume, for instance, what that creature was benefited from, and how the item is this way developed or matured! For instance, ParmigianoReggiano DOP is created in a little zone from the milk of explicit type of dairy animals as per customary techniques, and just cheddar that meets these particular criteria can be named and called ParmigianoReggiano DOP. Parmesan then again, is the general term applied to other comparative cheeses made outside that particular region and frequently outside Italy and as an impersonation of the genuine item. So it is imperative to remember this differentiation when shopping and understand the distinction in costs between the different items and likewise the distinction in quality and taste. DOP items are results of greater which have been sold at more significant expenses. Some DOP items which can be found outside Italy include ParmigianoReggiano, Prosciutto di Parma, Pecorino Toscano, AcetoBalsamicoTraditionale di Modena, and Mozzarella di Bufala.

IGP: IndicazioneGeographicaProtetta (Protected Geographical Indication). It applies to items that are explicit to a zone. However, they can be made with fixings from somewhere else. A portion of the IGP items is Lardo di Colonnala, the fix pork fat developed in unique marble bowls in Tuscany. The uncommon microclimate of the region and the techniques for generation give this item novel highlights, and the IGP assignment shields it from mediocre impersonations. The IGP assignment is regularly utilized for fruits, vegetables, and other products like the Lemons of

Sorrento, the porcino tomatoes of Sicily, the lentils of Umbria, which is all found on the Mediterranean Diet pyramid and can be utilized for any Mediterranean Diet food.

Numerous Italian items are customary of Italy and don't convey the DOP and IGP assignment, and yet they can be utilized to deliver true and top-notch Italian food. On the off chance that anyway, you are searching for valid quality investigate the DOP and IGP assignments.

Italian Cuisine is the cooking which can be discovered everywhere throughout the world. In practically every one of the towns of the world, you can locate a little or a huge Italian café or Pizza place. Italian food is the normal food in Italian and American homes as well as in homes everywhere throughout the world. And we are certain that you may discover bounty Italian foods and recipes which can fulfill your taste and want and keep you on track the healthy and wholesome Mediterranean diet.

Find out about the Job of Juice in your Healthy Mediterranean Diet

Juices bring the freshness and fitness of nature in our glass! Juices are not only for breakfast! We can make new and healthy, brimming with nutrients and different supplements, juices consistently from seasonal fruits, so we will appreciate them with our dinners as a stimulating beverage. Crisp juices are a piece of the Mediterranean Diet, and they are found in the high-recurrence step of the Mediterranean Diet pyramid. They are likely the most beneficial choice for competitors, and each one of the individuals who practice day by day.

Crisp Juices from new seasonal fruits have a significant and driving job in our present healthy diet because they are loaded with nutrients. Because of this significant dietary significance, juices are the partner of our body's wellbeing. You can appreciate juices every day and regularly as directed by the Mediterranean diet pyramid. Underneath, we will give you ten dietary tips for you to keep up great wellbeing.

Weight Loss: In a request for you to get more fit, you should have healthy and all-around adjusted suppers. You have to eat an assortment of suppers and foods to provide for your body the fundamental nutrients and different supplements which are required for every day exercises relying upon the phase of development and age you are in. The recurrence of every food, Mediterranean food, is given by the Mediterranean diet pyramid. The Med diet pyramid expresses that you ought to eat in any event two crisp fruits or one glass of new juice in the middle of dinners. Ensure that your suppers are finished in proteins, starches, nutrients, filaments, and other important components.

Diet Plan: You ought to change your week by week or month to month supper plan dependent on your day by day life as opposed to altering your day by day exercises around a diet plan. It is the best way to ensure that you pursue the diet plan when it depends on close to home daily schedule and exercises and around your working hours and breaks. You ought to adhere to the fundamental guideline, the standard of constant, and adjusted suppers. In your week after a week's diet plan, you should ensure that you remember new fruits and crisp juices for the request to have nature as your partner to guarantee and keep up wellbeing and wellbeing.

New Juices and fruits: Fresh fruits and juices have a main job in the Mediterranean diet since they contain the essential nutrients required for our body. Because of their significant dietary benefit, crisp juices establish the common partner of our wellbeing. They are the best decision for competitors and every one of the individuals who pay attention to working out. As we probably are aware, the Mediterranean diet isn't finished without visit physical exercise. A Mediterranean diet and physical are combined.

Eating propensities: We all realize that the "completion signal" lands from our stomach to the cerebrum around 10 minutes, some state 20 minutes, after the fact than the time our stomach is full. This implies on the off chance that we eat quickly we will eat a great deal of food which isn't important for us and which will most presumably be included/put away as fat in our body, prompting an overweight and stout body. We ought to subsequently eat gradually, so we will allow the correct sign to be given to the cerebrum. We ought to dedicate 10 minutes of our rest time to our supper time with the goal that we will appreciate the feast and, in this manner, set up the correct eating propensities. Bite well each nibble, appreciate the flavor of the food, its smell, and shading and drink your glass of wine, it is a piece of the Mediterranean diet, gradually. On the off chance that you can't drink wine, drink a healthy juice. Mediterranean diet is likewise about associating during a feast.

Fruits and Vegetables: If you are not as of now following the Mediterranean Diet, then we propose you include at any rate one organic product or vegetable in each feast. This is a great start for a decent and healthy diet, which will be the initial move towards the full appropriation of the Mediterranean diet. Ensure that fruits and vegetables are at a spot, you can have easy access, regardless of whether these are in your cooler or on your kitchen table. Gradually and step by step include one increasingly vegetable in your dinners. You may likewise attempt to make a mix of blended juices from fruits and vegetables, with the goal that you would exploit the healthful benefits of both fruits and vegetables.

Squeezed orange: Oranges are plentiful in Vitamin C, folic corrosive, potassium, selenium, filaments, carotene-b, iron, phosphorus, manganese, sodium, chlorine and Zinc. A glass of naturally pressed squeezed orange is a perfect segment of the Mediterranean diet breakfast. It offers to your body the essential vitality so it would adapt to the day's demands while simultaneously it gives a lot of the nutrients required for your day by day needs.

Exercise: Half an hour of vigorous exercise or 10,000 steps regularly are viewed as enough for the upkeep of good health and to keep the weight of the body at ordinary levels. We can achieve everything and anything we need by making straightforward and solid strides as long as we love our selves and deal with them as merited. Our dietary propensities are day by day food utilization is the prescription to our body.

Sustaining fixings: In specific times of fasting or times of restricted food utilization, the requirements for the utilization of feeding fixings increments. Crisp juices, which are plentiful in nutrients and different follows, offer moment vitality to your body while they likewise spread a noteworthy level of the body's needs in fluids. You ought not to overlook that half of each glass of juice is an unadulterated fluid commitment to the body's needs

Excursions: During get-aways, we appreciate a few drinks, for example, grenadines, smoothies, and numerous others, which contain a lot of calories because these drinks contain significant levels of sugar or liquor. It would be better for us and our body to expend such drinks incidentally and as uncommon as could reasonably be expected. When on an extended get-away, we ought to remember for our drinks, water, and new blended juices. Blended juices contain the wholesome benefits of more than one fruit. The different mixes of fruits in the planning of juices guarantee a more noteworthy assortment of wholesome segments, for example, Vitamins and cancer prevention agents.

Healthy method for living: Regular exercise or normal cooperation in physical exercises and exercise classes will empower the utilization of numerous calories on a day by day level and, in this manner, increment your body's digestion while simultaneously advance your wellbeing as a rule. We generally start our activities in little steps, and we proceed by expanding the week after week practice time until we reach a feasible and reasonable level. You have to recollect that while you practice, you have to expend many fluids to keep up the correct fluid equalization in your body in order to maintain a strategic distance from lack of hydration, which may influence your presentation.

Note that whichever diet you choose to receive, crisp juices ought to be a piece of it. They are healthy and reviving, and they add to the fitness of the body and brain. The individuals of the Mediterranean Sea have perceived the benefits of juices, and they have not just received them as a component of their diet, the Mediterranean Diet. However, they have guaranteed that they are one of their days by day and most successive Mediterranean foods and drinks.

Healthy Mediterranean Diet Foods for all

Mediterranean Diet foods are those foods which are eaten by the individuals in the Mediterranean nations and are a piece of the Mediterranean Diet pyramid. We realize that the Mediterranean diet contains a lot of fruits and vegetables since they are found in the " most continuous" class of the Med diet pyramid. It additionally contains numerous different foods which are found in different classifications of the Med diet pyramid, and these are the foods that we will make reference to and dissect further down in this article so we will turn out to be increasingly acquainted with the

Mediterranean foods, grasp them, cook them and off-kilter eat them!

We as a whole realize that Mediterranean foods are healthy foods particularly and guarantee for our body's wellbeing particularly for our heart. Yet, we should be cautious when we take foods with high unsaturated fats because even though they are useful for our heart they can prompt weight increase due the expanded calorie consumption as the old Greeks used to state: "Pan metron Ariston", Everything in Moderation. So we have to adjust our diet and expend the essential segments.

So what are the Mediterranean diet foods? We will attempt to give the names and a significant level portrayal of a portion of the Mediterranean foods, some of which are known, and some might be new to a large portion of you. The Mediterranean cooking is outstanding for its freshness and wellbeing, and the Mediterranean diet recipes are various, and it is unquestionably troublesome if not difficult to list every one of them in one article. The key elements of Mediterranean food include Olive oil, vegetables, legumes, fish, eggs, and poultry. Olive oil, which is known for its properties against malignant growth is a fundamental fixing in each prepared food or Mediterranean salad. Olive oil is a piece of all the Mediterranean foods. The Mediterranean recipes are off base not finish without the essential Mediterranean herbs and flavors, which add flavor and taste to each food.

Grains in the Mediterranean were left foul, and they were utilized in this structure in numerous Mediterranean foods and really taking the shape of pasta, bread, and couscous. The fact that grains were utilized grungy positively affected the strength of the individuals since they were processed gradually, and subsequently, glucose was delivered increasingly slow assimilated simpler by the body. Likewise, grains held their fiber and Vitamin E in this manner, shielding us from different interminable diseases.

Since meat ought to be eaten once in a while in the Mediterranean diet, the Mediterranean individuals have discovered a substantial flavor substitute for it, and this is no other than the eggplant. It is a vegetable appropriate for suppers with sauces and one which has fiber and potassium while its skin has malignant growth battling properties.

Chickpeas have a place with the legumes family and are one of the foods which can be eaten every day. They give top-notch protein and are wealthy in fiber. There are numerous recipes around which have Chickpeas as their principle fixing, which implies that eating chickpeas day by day or each other day won't be a similar encounter. You can make a chickpeas dinner as the principle dish, you can utilize them in salads, or you make paddies out of them and heat them in the broiler. Whatever the case might be, legumes ought to be one of the foods which should have a steady and continuous job in your diet.

Fish is another steady food in the Mediterranean diet. The Mediterranean individuals have a great deal of fish in their diet since they live around the Mediterranean Sea. Each sort of fish is healthy and particularly the sleek ones which are rich in omega-3 unsaturated fats, which are helpful to our heart. Fish can be eaten flame-broiled or heated, plain, or in the mix of different sauces. Fish is a fundamental part of the Mediterranean diet, and you should attempt to eat however much like fish as could reasonably be expected

Another fundamental segment of the Mediterranean diet is nuts. Nuts are extremely gainful to the human body, and they are utilized as a fixing in numerous foods. They are utilized in numerous salads, and they are fixing, together with nectar, which may go with a

Greek yogurt nibble. The most well-known nuts utilized are almonds.

Greek yogurt is a piece of the dairy items family which are discovered the "every now and again eat" classification of the Mediterranean diet. Yogurt and white cheeses can and ought to be devoured much of the time since they are wealthy in Calcium and secure us against osteoporosis. There are many white pieces of cheese in the market that originate from different Mediterranean countries. We have the ricotta cheddar from Italy, Mato cheddar from Spain, the French Chevre cheddar, the Turkish BeyazPeynir, the Greek feta cheddar, and the Cypriot Halloumi cheddar.

As we have expressed before, all else, there are numerous recipes that have a few or the entirety of the Mediterranean Diet fixings. A portion of the well known Mediterranean diet dishes is the Greek Moussaka, which has eggplant and potato as its fundamental fixings. The Italian minestrone soup is a healthy soup that can keep you warm during the virus winter period. The Moroccan chicken with couscous has become extremely a famous dish everywhere throughout the world. A well known East-Mediterranean dish is falafel, which is made of fava beans or chickpeas. The rundown may continue forever, and the varieties are, as we frequently state, constrained by our creative mind.

How might you realize that you are cooking a Mediterranean diet dish? All things considered, one may state that each healthy dish is a Mediterranean diet dish; however, this is a distortion. The Mediterranean diet dishes have as their essential fixings the foods recorded in the Mediterranean diet pyramid, and they are cooked by the custom of the Mediterranean individuals. You ought not to neglect to utilize Mediterranean herbs and flavors in each dinner you make with the goal that you would include the important taste and smell to your dish. Herbs may substitute salt much of the time, and remember them for your recipes guarantees the correct mixing of fixings giving your Mediterranean food an alternate and absolutely prevalent measurement.

Mediterranean Drinks

Mediterranean Diet is a method for living that includes all parts of living: food, drinks, practicing, and mingling. At the point when we notice food, we as a whole, understand what we mean by Mediterranean foods and Mediterranean cooking. Be that as it may, when we notice Mediterranean Drinks, a few people may not understand what this classification may incorporate, and consequently, we will attempt to list various Mediterranean Drinks with the goal that we will give a wide understanding of this classification.

What sort of drinks goes under the Mediterranean Drinks classification? We will attempt to list the different customary and non-conventional Mediterranean drinks, so we will give you a more extensive image of the Mediterranean diet.

Water: Water is the most significant beverage of the Mediterranean diet. It is typically prescribed that every individual ought to have in any event eight glasses of water; the Mediterranean individuals accept that every individual should take in any event six glasses of water every day. Water goes with each Mediterranean feast, and it is a piece of the Mediterranean culture to have water on the table with each dinner. Water, as a rule, goes with each treatment, and it assuredly goes with espressos like the Greek or Turkish or Lebanese espresso.

Squeezed orange: Orange juice normally goes with the Mediterranean diet breakfast, but it very well may be expended at any occurrence and at each event. Oranges are created in wealth in the Mediterranean locale since the atmosphere is appropriate for their development, and they are expended from various perspectives: as a natural product, as a juice, in foods, in pastries and desserts. Oranges are plentiful in Vitamin C. One glass of squeezed orange has 39 calories and will give 71% of our every day needs in Vitamin C. We ought to consistently have as a top priority that we ought to devour a new squeezed orange quickly or with a limit of a little ways from the time it is crushed since a portion of its gainful supplements are lost or scattered after a time of introduction to the air. So have this as a top priority when you press oranges for a crisp squeezed orange with your Mediterranean diet breakfast.

Pomegranate Juice: Mediterranean Diet is wealthy in fruits and vegetables, and their utilization isn't constrained to simply the fruits; however, the fruits can be transformed into juices. One juice which is well known in the Mediterranean bowl is the pomegranate juice. Pomegranate is utilized in the Mediterranean cooking, and the pomegranate juice is served during lunch or supper, and it isn't just reviving throughout the mid-year days, yet it is likewise useful for our wellbeing. Pomegranate juice is famous in Turkey, and the Arab nations of the Mediterranean Sea, and you can discover it at each edge of huge towns. Pomegranate juice is plentiful in nutrient C Potassium is wealthy in dietary fiber, and it contains cell reinforcements keeping our body healthy and brimming with vitality.

Lemonade: Lemon is another product of the citrus family, which is full nutrients and is utilized for cooking and as an added substance to foods. Its juice can't be flushed by the vast majority as a crisply crushed juice, and consequently, local people, the Mediterranean individuals, have figured out how to appreciate it by creating lemonade. Lemonade is a beverage that can be found in the entirety of the Mediterranean nations, and in light of the fact that it very well may be protected for a significant stretch, it can be appreciated consistently, particularly during the long summer months. Lemonade is served in each Mediterranean house cold with the option of a mint leaf because you need to include an extraordinary reviving taste.

Ayran: Ayran is a virus drink produced using yogurt with the expansion of salt. It is a beverage that is well known in Turkey, Lebanon, Syria, Israel, Cyprus, and Greece. It is viewed as the national beverage of Turkey, and it is best smashed during the sweltering summer a very long time as a backup of Mediterranean lunch or supper. It is easy to make Ayran at home, and on the off chance that you have never smashed it, we suggest you attempt it throughout the late spring, and you will cherish it. All you have to make is yogurt, salt, and a few leaves of slashed mint, ideally dried mint. We need not advise you that yogurt and particularly Greek Yogurt is a piece of the Mediterranean diet.

Sahlep or Salep or Sahlap: Sahlep is a hot beverage that is tanked in the Mediterranean locale involved by the Ottoman Empire. The beverage is made by blending Sahlep flour with heated water or milk. Sahlep flour is produced using Orchids plants. It is an extremely delectable, conventional, warming, and invigorating beverage of the eastern Mediterranean area, and it is known as the beverage of Turkey.

Almond Drink, Soumada: This almond drink is a customary Greek beverage which is produced using almonds, sweet and severe. Soumada is generally served during upbeat events because of its white shading, and such events are weddings. In some different locales of the Mediterranean, similar to Cyprus, Soumada is smashed warm, giving the glow and decent smell of almonds. This is another approach to appreciate the health benefits of almonds.

Pepitada: Pepitada is a beverage produced using the simmered/toasted seeds of the melons. It has its own unmistakable taste and smell, and it is a customary beverage among the Jewish people group of Greece since it is the beverage that is utilized to break the Yom Kippur quick. It is a heavenly drink, easy to make, and its shading and immaculateness are the reasons it has been chosen to be tanked during this significant Jewish occasion.

Tea: Tea is a beverage delighted in by numerous Mediterranean countries, particularly those countries which were a piece of the Ottoman Empire. Tea is a beverage that needs no presentation, and it is currently viewed as a world beverage instead of a Mediterranean beverage since the British have spread it all through the world.

Espresso: You will discover numerous varieties of espresso in the Mediterranean locale. There is the French espresso, the Italian coffee or cappuccino, the Greek espresso, the Turkish espresso, the Lebanese espresso, and the Egyptian espresso. The last four are varieties of what was known as the Ottoman espresso. Espresso is tanked for the duration of the day, and it is positively part of the Mediterranean breakfast or a beverage that is smashed after a decent lunch. It is served in the different customary coffeehouses of the Mediterranean, and it is a beverage offered to visitors when they visit companions or family members.

Wine: Wine is a piece of the Mediterranean diet. A glass of wine as a component of lunch or supper is suggested by numerous specialists and dieticians. The helpful impacts of wine have been perceived during the time by the old Greeks and later on by the Romans.A glass of red wine for lunch or supper is an absolute necessity in specific nations like France, Italy, and Greece. Wine enables our body to battle particular kinds of disease and has cancer prevention agent properties.

Sangria: Sangria is a Spanish beverage comprising of wine, slashed fruits, sugar, and some brandy or cognac.

It is a beverage that has gotten famous all around the globe, and it consolidates the benefits of the wine and the fruits, which are a significant segment of the Mediterranean diet.

The rundown of the Mediterranean drinks may continue endlessly, as the Mediterranean human advancements have been around for thousands of years, and the Mediterranean diet has been their method for the living of an equivalent period. Mediterranean drinks and foods structure the Mediterranean cooking, and all are a piece of the Mediterranean diet.

Mediterranean Diet Recipes foods for a Healthy Lunch

We have talked about the significance of the Mediterranean Diet breakfast, and we have given you a few thoughts of what individuals in the Mediterranea district have for breakfast. As everyone recognizes, breakfast is the most significant supper of the day. You need to have breakfast like a lord, the state. Be that as it may, you can't have a healthy and lively day with only one supper. You have to give your body the fundamental fuel on a regular premise. So need a healthy Mediterranean diet lunch. The Mediterranean diet lunch food will be your second feast of the day and needs to increase the value of the effectively taken Mediterranean breakfast.

There are truly thousands of recipes and thoughts for a healthy Mediterranean lunch. What is useful for the Mediterranean individuals is beneficial for you also. The significant thing is to have a fair diet, and so as to accomplish this, you have to plan for it. It is valid for what they state that in the event that you don't have a plan, any street will take you there! As we have referenced ordinarily, it is critical to have a month to month or a week after week diet plan with the goal that you and your family would realize what to look for cooking and what you will have for lunch, since we as a whole concur that the Mediterranean diet is useful for the whole family.

So what are a portion of the Mediterranean diet foods and recipes for a decent, nourishing, and healthy lunch? We will attempt to portray an assortment of foods and recipes from various nations of the Mediterranean district with the goal that you will get a more extensive understanding of the significance of lunch in these nations and at the same time pick what is best for you and your family, in view of your taste and inclinations.

Mediterranean Tuna salad is a phenomenal and easy thought for lunch. In the event that you love to fish, you have to maintain a strategic distance from the mainstream and yet unhealthy fish salad with mayonnaise. There are numerous recipes around, which use fish with numerous other Mediterranean foods found in the Mediterranean diet pyramid-like, cappers, tomatoes, olive oil, and olives.

Greek Salad is another alternative for lunch since the Greek salad is accessible at numerous eateries as a side dish or starter as well as a principal dish too. What are the elements of a Greek salad? Nothing else except for new vegetables like cucumbers, tomatoes, onion, olives, and feta cheddar. Olive oil is another fundamental fixing, and there is no compelling reason to help you to remember the benefits of olive oil and the fact that it battles malignancy! From a healthful perspective, you have to realize that cucumbers are a portion of food with low calories and high in nutrient K. They likewise have a sufficient amount of Vitamin C, and thus they are now and then alluded to as the superfood of the Mediterranean diet.

Mediterranean recipes with couscous are additionally another well-known lunch thought. A mainstream couscous formula is a couscous with chickpeas and almonds. Couscous is a customary Moroccan dish, and it regularly thought to be a grain item while it is really a pasta item! One cup of couscous has around 176 calories, zero immersed fats, and a decent level of starches required for your day by day utilization. You can likewise make decent salads utilizing Couscous as the fundamental fixing.

Pasta is another incredible choice for a fast and healthy Mediterranean food for lunch. Traditionally, Italian dish, pasta, can be found wherever on the planet, and you need not be reminded that Italian food was positioned as the main of the best ten cooking styles of the world! Pasta can be presented with any sort of tomato sauce which can be joined with fish and/or vegetables and different Mediterranean herbs. The varieties and mixes for a pasta dish are various and practically endless, and hence we will leave your creative mind to ad-lib. If you are making lunch, all you need is a bit of planning in order to have the correct fixings at home.

A fish and seafood lunch is another phenomenal thought for a healthy lunch. You can have a barbecued trout or squid with bubbled vegetables and consequently get quite a few supplements you should proceed with your day. Fish and seafood are found in the incessant class of the Mediterranean diet, and they can be eaten 1-2 times each week. You may discover crisp fish at your closest store or fish market, and you can cook it in different manners utilizing a few Mediterranean diet herbs and flavors to include the correct flavor and evacuate the fishy smell a portion of the fish have. One of my top choices is the Octopus meal.

Vegetable snacks are likewise well known in the Mediterranean area. Legumes are in the high use step of the Mediterranean pyramid, and it is proposed that you have day by day or practically every day. You can include them in salads or cook them and serve them as fundamental dish went with different vegetables, for example, spinach and hacked scallions. An extremely well-known center eastern plunge is Humus produced using chickpeas. In the event that you allude to any Mediterranean diet cookbook, you will discover many thoughts regarding vegetable-based snacks.

This is off-kilter a facetious inquiry since it is realized that the Spanish individuals give a great deal of accentuation on food, and consequently, they are known as the foodies of Europe! So what is an average Spanish dish for lunch? Gazpacho soup and Paellaare only two of the most famous dishes for a decent and healthy Mediterranean diet lunch, and they are exceptionally wholesome too.

In the event that you extravagant a burger for lunch, you may have one as long as you don't damage the recurrence rules of the pyramid. You can have a chicken or a turkey burger rather than a meat burger, and you should assuredly keep away from singed potatoes by having broiler cooked fries. You may likewise join your burger with a decent new vegetable salad.

As you may have just made sense of, the choices and mixes for a healthy Mediterranean lunch as various, and they are just restricted by your taste and craving. You can search for any Mediterranean diet formula, in the event that you are in the mind-set for cooking, or you may search for a Mediterranean diet café close to you, with the goal that you will appreciate a healthy and dietary Mediterranean Diet lunch. Recollect that you have to have lunch like a Prince.

Mediterranean Breakfast or Mediterranean Diet Breakfast

Regularly we are found out about the Mediterranean breakfast, and then in the following magazine or at the following online journal, we run over the

Mediterranean Diet breakfast, and we are attempting to understand the distinction. Is there are contrast? Truly and No. Everything depends on what direction you take a gander at it. We will attempt to investigate the two and give you the genuine benefits of the Mediterranean Diet breakfast. In the more seasoned occasions, there was no genuine distinction between the two.

In exacting terms, Mediterranean breakfast is the morning meal Mediterranean individuals have during their regular day to day existence, and it could possibly be healthy. We ought not to imagine that a morning meal taken in the Mediterranean bowl is constantly healthy and nourishing. It might happen to be that individuals eat frankfurters and bacon and eggs each day, and they might be living in Italy or Spain. Does this make it a healthy breakfast? No, unquestionably not. It is anyway a Mediterranean breakfast since wiener is delicacy produce of numerous

Mediterranean nations, yet they are in the "less frequently" classification of the Med diet pyramid. Additionally, eggs are a piece of the Mediterranean diet, and in the Mediterranean Diet pyramid, they can be found in the "moderate to week by week" segment of the pyramid. So as you may have just construed eating eggs and bacon or hotdogs isn't healthy in any way, however, if you have them once in a while, state more than once per month, at that point there ought to be no issue.

The Mediterranean Diet breakfast anyway is something entirely unexpected. It is the morning meal which is devoured toward the beginning of the day by the individuals who pursue the Mediterranean Diet and may live at any piece of the world, from California to Australia and from Chile to China. So what can a Mediterranean diet breakfast be? It can comprise of fruits and vegetables, nuts, whole grain oats and bread, olives, tomatoes. It very well may be, on a less regular period, yogurt and other dairy items, and it can even be eggs and frankfurters, yet this must be on more than one occasion per month. You should adjust your morning meal, eat different foods, and pursue the Mediterranean Diet pyramid to decide the utilization recurrence. We certainly bolster the planning of week by week or even a month to month eating plan, which will empower you to screen what you and your family eat and guarantee that a dietary equalization plan is pursued. Setting up a dietary plan is easy, and it tends to be a family issue joined with fun! Recollect that on the off chance that you include your family into this, at that point, they are bound to pursue the Med diet.

Breakfast ought to be the most extravagant feast of the day. It is the dinner that will prop you up the whole day and will awaken your body and psyche with the goal that you will adapt for the remainder of the day. Nonetheless, most extravagant doesn't mean the heaviest supper of the day. Breakfast ought not to make you awkward and ought not to force on your stomach, requiring substantial exercises for absorption. You need the blood for the remainder of your body and your cerebrum. A decent breakfast ought to be wealthy in strands and filaments are contained in fruits and whole-grain items. You may likewise remember dried fruits and nuts for your grain breakfast. A decent breakfast should comprise of foods which are low in fats. So you have to maintain a strategic distance from red meats and bacon! A decent Mediterranean diet breakfast might be wealthy in omega-3 unsaturated fats, which implies it might comprise, in full or to some extent, with seafood like smoked salmon.

A decent Mediterranean diet breakfast should consider the dietary propensities and requirements of the family, the season, and the land area of the individual having it. A healthy and wholesome breakfast ought to fulfill the requirements of the relatives. Elderly individuals have unexpected needs in comparison to children, and individuals who are experiencing constant diseases like Diabetes ought to devour the correct foods. Individuals experiencing a cold or influenza may pick a morning meal more extravagant in Vitamin C and consequently, remember for their morning meal Citrus fruits and citrus juices. A Mediterranean diet breakfast is constantly balanced, dependent on the season. Since a rich Mediterranean diet breakfast comprises of fruits and vegetables, we utilize the fruits and vegetables which are in season to set up our morning meal. Utilizing fruits and vegetables which are in season bodes well since they are crisp and less expensive than some other options. Picking seasonal fruits and vegetables empowers you to have the ideal variety in our everyday diet and make the correct incitements. Likewise, your body has various needs throughout the winter than in the mid-year, so seasonal foods stregnthen your body to change in accordance with the distinctive ecological conditions. Land areas force the utilization of various fixings, flavors, and herbs for the arrangement of your morning meal. You should attempt to use it. However, much neighborhood produces as could reasonably be expected. For example, when you are in Spain, you may utilize Mato cheddar for your morning meal while when in Turkey, you are well on the way to utilize the BeyazPeynir white cheddar.

There are truly thousands of Mediterranean Diet breakfast recipes that can fulfill any taste and any need. There basic and quick breakfast recipes, and there are more perplexing and tedious ones who are there to fulfill the most demanding Med diet devotees. You may have a basic Greek Yogurt breakfast with dried fruits and nuts which are accessible in your kitchen, or you might need to have a goat cheddar filled the crepe with walnuts and nectar. However you take a gander at it, it ought to be a fair breakfast which will top you off and give you the correct vitality to prop you up till the whole day.

The Mediterranean Diet breakfast ought to be your greatest and most extravagant supper of the day, and it ought to be a really Mediterranean breakfast! It ought not to be a similar breakfast all day every day and should comprise of crisp produce, wealthy in fiber, which is in season. Adhere to these straightforward guidelines joined with a 30-40 mins physical exercise, and you will have a healthy body and psyche since a physical exercise some portion of the Mediterranean Diet.

What do you hope to discover in a Mediterranean diet basic food item list?

What do you hope to discover in a Mediterranean diet basic food item list? This isn't an inquiry that is of worry to the Mediterranean diet supporters! Drug diet devotees realize that when they go to the basic food item shop, they will shop new and healthy items, which will empower them to cook their preferred Mediterranean foods for breakfast, lunch, or supper.

We as a whole know, as Mediterranean diet adherents, that we are not on any weight loss program, and we are not on any hardship program either. We have received and pursue a healthy method for leaving dependent on a demonstrated diet, the Mediterranean Diet, which has been the diet of numerous countries and nationalities over the span of history. Mediterranean Diet has not been designed by somebody with the point of selling an item or help, and it is just advanced intentionally by individuals who trust in this diet with the sole motivation behind making this diet known to the remainder of the world.

One significant parameter concerning our staple rundown is that by following the Mediterranean diet, we are eating more advantageous as well as we set aside cash also!! Off-kilter, you may ask: how is this conceivable? This is on the grounds that in your mind, you have related modest food with inexpensive food, which is unquestionably not healthy.

The Mediterranean Diet staple rundown

Assembling a basic food item list relies upon numerous factors. It relies upon factors like: regardless of whether you work or not, whether you cook each supper from the day preceding or the time you are going to eat it, for what number of people you cook, and so forth. The ideal approach to handle a staple rundown is by planning, and so as to do this, you need a printed or an electronic rundown of the things you generally shop. Utilizing the rundown, you may check what you have available and what you have to purchase. The subject obviously might be, for what number of dinners do I plan and hence shop?

Typically individuals plan the suppers of the week having as a primary concern a decent, from all perspectives, feast plan put together off-kilter with respect to the Mediterranean Diet pyramid and the recurrence with which you can eat particular kinds of food. It's implied that the crisp fruits and vegetables can be and ought to be a piece of your day by day suppers and bites. Your feast plan can be planned on a week after week premise and may have certain characteristics like Kid-accommodating on the off chance that it is a supper the children love, veggie-lover, quick or superfast on the off chance that it is a dinner you can make rapidly, fish supper in the event that it depends on fish and so forth. Another ascribe to be considered when planning for the suppers is the number of calories every segment of our feast has. You may allude to different books or online records about the number of calories every feast segment has, and you can act as needs be. It ought to be noted here that once you pursue the Mediterranean diet, you eat respectably and practice consistently you ought not to stress over calories since the Med diet continuously drives you to a healthy body with a typical and healthy Body Mass Index, BMI.

Exceptional consideration ought to be taken when setting up the basic food item list for individuals who have any sort of incessant diseases like Diabetes, Heart issues, or for individuals with Muscular dystrophy or comparative sort of diseases. Studies have demonstrated that the Mediterranean diet helps individuals who experience the ill effects of different diseases, yet the basic food item rundown ought to be balanced in like manner.

What is advisable for you to remember for your Grocery list?

As we probably are aware, the Mediterranean diet is wealthy in fruits, vegetables, fish, whole grain oat, dairy items, and other healthy foods ate less every now and again, for example, white meat. So when you go out for staple goods, your basic food item rundown ought to incorporate all the recently referenced foods however in various amounts relying upon the week by week plan, which was readied.

Whole Grains: Your shopping rundown should incorporate whole grain foods, whole grain oat, and/or whole-grain bread. Whole grains are a piece of the regularly eat classification of the Mediterranean diet. Whole-grain foods take more time to process furnishing your body with all the healthy supplements. In the event, that whole grain foods are costly in your close by staple, and you might need to visit a wholesale store and store for seven days as well as maybe for the month.

Vegetables: Vegetables are a piece of the Mediterranean diet, and you should shop and cook vegetables which are in season as they are normally less expensive than others. In the event that anyway you want or plan to eat vegetables which are not in season, and you think of them as costly, try not to be reluctant to utilize solidified vegetables yet not canned food.

The facts demonstrate that solidified vegetables lose a portion of their dietary benefit; however, they are far superior to canned vegetables.

Fish: You should incorporate at any rate one fish feast in your week by week supper plan. Fish is a fundamental part of the Mediterranean diet. Fish are wealthy in omega-3 cancer prevention agents, and there is an extraordinary assortment of fish to suit each taste and want. You can cook only it or with pasta, barbecued or in the stove. You ought to stay away from singed fish.

Olive oil: Your basic food item rundown should incorporate olive oil and olives. You can utilize olive oil as a salad dressing or for your cooking. The advantageous impacts of olive oil are notable and all around recorded by numerous investigations.

White meats: If your week by week plan incorporates meat, it should be white meat. You may have red meat once a month, yet white meat like poultry or Turkey can be devoured once every week. You can pick solidified meats if your financial limit can't take care of the expense of crisp white meat.

Cheddar: Cheese is much of the time utilized in the Mediterranean diet. White cheddar is in the week by week utilization list while the more adult yellow cheddar ought to devour less much of the time, yet it is still alright to be expended.

Yogurt: Low-fat yogurt is a piece of the Mediterranean diet, and on the off chance that you like to yogurt, you should change to Greek Yogurt as it has expanded benefits, and it more beneficial with fewer calories than other sorts of yogurts. So your basic food item rundown ought to incorporate Greek yogurt for the whole family as yogurt can be had as breakfast, some portion of your lunch, or as a tidbit.

You should do the shopping for food fun, and this can be positively accomplished by ordering your Mediterranean Diet Grocery list with the whole family and picking foods, fruits, and vegetables, which will be eaten by all. When you aggregate and go through a few staple records, you will understand that your excursion to the Grocery store is fun and intriguing since you will become familiar with a ton and you will going through all the healthy food segments of the store, and you will smell the new fruits and vegetables.

Mediterranean Recipes

The Mediterranean diet is stacked with vegetables, fruits, legumes, whole grains, and olive oil. Literally adjusting to a Mediterranean diet is probably the most advantageous decision you can make for yourself.

What is a Mediterranean Diet Recipe?

Mediterranean recipes joined with the Mediterranean diet put accentuation on eating essentially plant-based foods, for example, swhole grains, vegetables, and fruits, nuts, and legumes.

Couple these things with healthy fats and supplant salt with vigorous herbs and flavors to season food. In the event that you are eating Mediterranean food to get healthy, limit your red meat admission to close to a couple of times each month and eat poultry and fish, at any rate, two times per week.

In the event that your PCP gives you the approval, you can even have a glass of red or white wine to a great extent.

What foods to eat and not to Eat on the Mediterranean diet?

In the event that simply beginning on the Mediterranean diet, you may have a few inquiries. Because you wind up thinking about what you ought to and shouldn't eat, you are not the only one.

Eat Vegetables, fruits, nuts, seeds, legumes, potatoes, whole grains, pieces of bread, herbs, flavors, fish, seafood, and additional virgin olive oil.

Eat with some restraint: Poultry, eggs, cheddar, and yogurt.

Try not to eat: Sugar-improved refreshments, included sugars, prepared meat, refined grains, refined oils, and other exceptionally handled foods.

The Mediterranean diet is centered around an assortment of healthy food things, constraining the not all that healthy one.

Mediterranean food isn't just a delectable and healthy approach to eat. However, it gives a few choices for you to browse with regards to hors d'oeuvres, salads, and even primary courses. Pick this flavourful method to appreciate a healthy and tasty feast each night of the week.

Easy Mediterranean Recipes

There are a large number of various Mediterranean motivated hors d'oeuvres to look over. Extending from things like Olive Hummus and Greek Gyro Nachos to

Spanakopita Tarts and Three Mushroom Pecorino Truffled Flatbread. There is an easy and healthy hors d'oeuvre for everybody.

MEDITERRANAEAN DIET RECIPES

Hors d'oeuvres

Straightforward Mediterranean Olive Oil Pasta

Mediterranean olive oil pasta is course reading Mediterranean diet heavenliness! It skirts all the lighten and overwhelming sauces for additional virgin olive oil and a couple of fixings.

This straightforward olive oil pasta formula takes motivation from a Naples dish called "spaghetti Aglio e olio. Or, "spaghetti with garlic and oil."

In a run of the mill spaghetti Aglio e olio formula, pasta is covered in a straightforward garlic-olive oil sauce, at that point decorated with parsley and ground Parmesan.

Be that as it may, this Mediterranean olive oil pasta goes only somewhat further by including a couple of most loved fixings like grape tomatoes, marinated artichoke hearts, feta, and olives.

Two or three tips for this olive oil pasta

To begin with, this dish makes a component of additional virgin olive oil and depends vigorously on its flavor. The oil is quickly warmed through, however not cooked. That is the reason, and you'll need to utilize the best quality additional virgin olive oil you can manage.

Keep in mind, oils that are essentially marked "unadulterated" have as a rule been heat-treated and refined by mechanical methods and, therefore, need character and flavor.

Early Harvest Extra Virgin Olive Oil

For this formula, I generally utilize our Greek Early Harvest additional virgin olive oil. It is naturally developed and prepared from local Koroneiki olives, which are hand-picked right off the bat in the season while still green, and handled inside our own to make this prized 'fluid gold' they call 'agoureleo.'

Our Early Harvest oil is a dazzling virus extricated and unfiltered oil with a consummately adjusted multifaceted nature-rich green, fruity, and impactful with a peppery completion. Our oil includes especially significant levels of polyphenols and low corrosiveness of under 0.35%.

Also, when causing the sauce to don't enable the garlic to darker, it will pollute its flavor. In the event that it browns or consumes, you'll have to hurl it and begin once again.

DESCRIPTION

Straightforward, delicious olive oil pasta stacked with Mediterranean flavors.

INGREDIENTS

- ❖ 1 lb slim spaghetti
- ❖ 1/2 cup Early Harvest Greek Extra Virgin Olive Oil (or Private Reserve Extra Virgin Olive Oil)
- ❖ Four garlic cloves, squashed
- ❖ Salt
- ❖ 1 cup hacked new parsley
- ❖ 12 oz grape tomatoes, split
- ❖ 3 scallions (green onions), top cut, the two whites, and greens hacked
- ❖ 1 tsp dark pepper
- ❖ 6 oz marinated artichoke hearts, depleted
- ❖ 1/4 cup set olives, split
- ❖ 1/4 cup disintegrated feta cheddar, more in the event that you like
- ❖ 10–15 new basil leaves, torn
- ❖ Zest of 1 lemon

❖ Crushed red pepper chips, discretionary

INSTRUCTIONS

1. Follow bundle instructions to cook slim spaghetti pasta to still somewhat firm (mine took 6 minutes to cook in a lot of bubbling water with salt and olive oil).

2. When pasta is nearly cooked, heat the additional virgin olive oil in an enormous cast-iron skillet over medium warmth. Lower the warmth and include garlic and a touch of salt. Cook for 10 seconds, blending routinely. Mix in the parsley, tomatoes, and slashed scallions. Cook over low warmth until simply warmed through, around 30 seconds, or somewhere in the vicinity.

3. When the pasta is prepared, expel from heat, channel cooking water, and come back to its cooking pot. Pour the warmed olive oil sauce in and hurl to cover completely. Include dark pepper and hurl again to cover.

4. Add the rest of the ingredients and hurl once again. Serve promptly in pasta bowls, and on the off chance that you like, top each with more basil leaves and feta. Appreciate!

Easy Homemade Chicken Shawarma

Where the avenues are loaded up with little stands and joints selling flavorful, overly fragrant Middle Eastern foods. Crisp singed falafel. Sticks of Kabobs. And indeed, shawarma, both hamburger, and chicken alternatives.

Chicken shawarma is one of my supreme most loved Middle Eastern road foods. You may or not be comfortable with it, so we should begin with what is chicken shawarma.

What is Chicken Shawarma?

Customary chicken shawarma is fundamentally well-marinated chicken, layered on a vertical rotisserie or spit where it's moderately simmered for a considerable length of time in its very own juices and fat—until impeccably delicate and extra delightful! To serve it, the joint proprietor would regularly shave a layer of shawarma off the spit and heap it up into a pita pocket, jazz it with tahini sauce, and tons of new garnishes!

I'm letting you know, and Chicken shawarma is the encapsulation of tempting Middle Eastern flavors. And the uplifting news is, I've discovered an easy method to make it at home with the equivalent real flavors.

For my easy custom made chicken shawarma variant, you needn't bother with an extraordinary rotisserie or spit. You simply need a sheet skillet to make it directly in the stove!

The mystery is in the shawarma zest blend, including warm flavors including cumin, coriander, turmeric, paprika, and a touch of cayenne. SO MUCH FLAVOR!

The Effective method to make chicken shawarma at home (Step-by-Step)

1. Make the shawarma flavor blend. Basically, include the flavors into a little bowl and blend to join.

2. Slice some boneless, skinless chicken thighs into little reduced down pieces (you can utilize chicken bosom on the off chance that you like, this is only my own inclination.)

3. Zest the chicken up, make a point to cover the chicken well with the zest blend. Include onions, lemon juice, and additional virgin olive oil. fOn the off chance that you have the opportunity, cover and refrigerate for 3 hours or medium-term (ifyou don't, you can skirt the marinating time, despite everything it'll be scrumptious)

4. At the point when prepared, lay the chicken shawarma on a huge sheet skillet and heat in 425 degrees warmed stove for 30 minutes or somewhere in

the vicinity (you can check somewhat prior as broilers do differ.)

How to Serve Chicken Shawarma?

The genuine Middle Eastern approach to serve chicken shawarma is in pita pockets or wraps with loads of veggies and a decent arrangement of sauce. I like stacked pita pockets.

Similarly, as with meat shawarma, you can serve chicken shawarma with a liberal sprinkle of tahini sauce. It's likewise regular to utilize a white yogurt-based sauce like Greek Tzatziki.

This chicken shawarma formula can serve 4 to 6 individuals. As it is, in case you're searching for a fun method to serve a bigger group, consider doing shawarma sliders.

Would you be able to make this shawarma ahead of time?

Indeed, you can plan and heat the chicken early a couple of evenings ahead of time and then amass into pita pockets when the opportunity arrives. Refrigerate in the tight-top holder until prepared to utilize.

DESCRIPTION

You needn't bother with an exceptional rotisserie to make this easy custom made chicken shawarma formula! Chicken pieces, hurled in warm Middle Eastern flavors, at that point heated until splendidly delicate. Make certain to look at the video and step-by-step above.

INGREDIENTS

- ❖ 3/4 tbsp ground cumin
- ❖ 3/4 tbsp turmeric powder
- ❖ 3/4 tbsp ground coriander
- ❖ 3/4 tbsp garlic powder
- ❖ 3/4 tbsp paprika
- ❖ 1/2 tsp ground cloves
- ❖ 1/2 tsp cayenne pepper, more in the event that you like

- ❖ Salt
- ❖ 8 boneless, skinless chicken thighs
- ❖ 1 huge onion, daintily cut
- ❖ 1 huge lemon, juice of
- ❖ 1/3 cup Private Reserve additional virgin olive oil

To Serve

- ❖ 6 pita pockets
- ❖ Tahini sauce or Greek Tzatziki sauce
- ❖ Baby arugula
- ❖ 3-fixing Mediterranean Salad
- ❖ Pickles or kalmata olives (discretionary)

INSTRUCTIONS

1. In a small bowl, blend the cumin, turmeric, coriander, garlic powder, sweet paprika, and cloves. Put aside the shawarma zest blend until further notice.

2. Pat the chicken thighs dry and seasoned it with salt on the two sides, daintily cut into little reduced down pieces.

3. Place the chicken in a huge bowl. Including the shwarma flavors and hurl to cover. With the onions, lemon juice, and olive oil. Cover and refrigerate for 3 hours or medium-term.

4. When prepared, pre-heat the stove to 425 degrees F. Remove the chicken from the cooler and let it sit at a normal room temperature for a couple of moments.

5. Spread the marinated chicken and the onions in a single layer, gently oiled preparing sheet skillet. Broil it for 30 minutes in the 425 degrees F warmed stove. For a progressively sautéed, crispier chicken, move the dish to the top rack and cook quickly (observe cautiously). Expel from the stove.

6. While the chicken is cooking, prepare the pita pockets. Make tahini sauce as indicated by this formula or Tzatziki sauce as per this formula. Make 3-fixing Mediterranean salad as per this formula. Put in a safe spot.

7. To serve it, open pita pockets up and then Spread a little tahini sauce or Tzatziki sauce, include chicken shawarma, arugula, Mediterranean salad and pickles or olives, if you like. Serve right away!

NOTES

•**Cook's Tip**: Marinate the chicken for 3 hours or medium-term in the ice chest. Else, you can skirt the marinating time as demonstrated in the instructions. It will at present, be delightful!

• Cook's Tip: Because stoves change, make certain to check chicken at around 25 minutes or so of simmering/heating and go from that point. Chicken is prepared when interior temperature arrives at 165 degrees F.

• Make-Ahead Option: You can set up the chicken early, a couple of evenings ahead of time, on the off chance that you like. Warm-up in a skillet over medium warmth, including a tad of fluid and hurling the chicken pieces until warmed through. Collect pita pockets as trained.

• **Serving Ideas:** The Chicken shawarma is best served in pita pockets with salad and sauces, similar to I referenced as of now, yet it very well may be filled in as a starter to a bigger group. All things considered, you can serve it in littler slider buns with only a little sauce and crisp arugula.

Greek Tzatziki Sauce Recipe

Tzatziki sauce formula it originated from the Greek island of Paros, where Stella Leonetti serves it routinely in her eatery called Rafeletti. Out of this world bona fide, however, I've pared it down a piece to meet my little family's requirements.

This is extraordinary and rich tzatziki with three-star ingredients: Greek yogurt, cucumber, and garlic.

A couple of significant tips for best outcomes

1-To make tzatziki, start by grinding the cucumber in your food processor with a spot of legitimate salt. I like to utilize English seedless cucumbers that have been in any event, in part, stripped. Ensure that you channel the cucumbers very well over a working strainer. You can do this step early, or in case you're in a surge, it's useful to put the ground cucumber in a spotless kitchen fabric or an overwhelming napkin and press all the fluid out.

2-I like to blend my genuine tzatziki sauce by hand in a huge bowl. Initially, join the garlic with white vinegar, additional virgin olive oil, and a squeeze progressively salt. Include the depleted cucumber. At long last, mix in the stressed yogurt (I utilize without fat Greek yogurt, yet the first formula calls for full-fat Greek yogurt.) Make sure to mix until everything is all around consolidated.

3-For best taste and surface spread tzatziki sauce firmly and refrigerate for two or three hours before use.

4-If you don't know you can handle this much garlic, start with a large portion of the measure of garlic the first occasion when you attempt it.

5-To switch things up, don't hesitate to mix shortly of new dill or mint (around 1 tablespoon or so ought to be adequate.)

Approaches to Use Tzatziki

The tzatziki sauce is adaptable; there are such huge numbers of approaches to appreciate it. For an easy hors d'oeuvre or nibble, I love to serve Tzatziki with warm bread and cut vegetables. Be that as it may, it makes an ideal fixing for Mediterranean-style prepared potato; or by stuffed snapper or dish seared trout; sheep slashes; chicken souvlaki; shawarma and more! I likewise use it essentially as a sandwich spread.

Make ahead and Storage Instructions

You can make tzatziki sauce early. It's ideal for storing it in the ice chest in a firmly secured glass holder. Use it inside 2 to 4 days.

DESCRIPTION

Rich Greek Tzatziki Sauce. A versatile Greek yogurt and cucumber sauce to serve alongside veggies and pita spread on sandwiches, or add it by flame-broiled fish, meat or poultry!

INGREDIENTS

- ❖ 3/4 English cucumber, somewhat stripped (striped) and cut
- ❖ 1 tsp genuine salt, separated
- ❖ 4 to 5 garlic cloves, stripped, finely ground or minced (you can utilize less in the event that you like)
- ❖ 1 tsp white vinegarr
- ❖ 1 tabsp Early Harvest Greek Extra Virgin Olive Oil
- ❖ 2 cups Greek yogurt (I utilized natural fat-free Greek yogurt, yet you can utilize 2% or whole milk Greek yogurt, in the event that you like)
- ❖ 1/4 tsp ground white pepper
- ❖ Warm pita bread for serving
- ❖ Sliced vegetables for serving

INSTRUCTIONS

1. Prep the cucumber. In a food processor, grind the cucumbers. Hurl with 1/2 tsp fit salt. Move to a fine work strainer over a profound bowl to deplete. Spoon the ground cucumber into a cheddar fabric or a

twofold thickness napkin and crush dry. Put aside quickly.

2. In one enormous blending bowl, place the garlic with staying 1/2 tsp salt, white vinegar, and additional virgin olive oil. Blend to consolidate.

3. Add the ground cucumber to the enormous bowl with the garlic blend. Mix in the yogurt and white pepper. Consolidate completely. Spread firmly and refrigerate for several hours.

4. When prepared to serve, mix the tzatziki sauce to revive and move to a serving bowl, sprinkle with all the more additional virgin olive oil, in the event that you like. Include a side of warm pita bread and your preferred vegetables. (additionally, observe notes for more thoughts)

NOTES

1. This formula is adjusted from Yogurt Culture. It is my fast form, and it's been chopped down to suit a little family.

2. Cook's Tips: This is a very garlicky plunge, in the event that you like, start with a little measure of garlic and fuse more varying. And to switch things up, don't hesitate to mix in a tablespoon or so of hacked new dill or crisp mint.

3. To Store: It's ideal for storing tzatziki in the refrigerator in a firmly secured glass holder, and use inside 2 to 4 days.

4. Suggestions for Use: Tzatziki makes the ideal fixing for Mediterranean-style prepared potato; or by stuffed snapper or container seared trout; sheep slashes; chicken souvlaki; shawarma and more! I likewise use it basically like a sandwich spread.

One-skillet Mediterranean Baked Halibut Recipe with Vegetables

Halibut Fish

Halibut is one of my preferred white fish to prepare. It is firm yet flaky and has a heartier, delicate surface than other white fish choices. And in case you're not enthusiastic about the flavor of fish, you would almost certainly value its gentle, somewhat sweet taste, which makes it an extraordinary candidate for a wide range of seasonings and flavors!

There are a large number of approaches to planning halibut–flame-broiled, seared, poached in a wine sauce (mmm so great), or basically heated like we have today.

Tip for purchasing halibut: If you're going for new halibut at your general store, ensure it looks white with a glossy tissue — Dodge dark-colored spots on the white substance. I realized as of late that 80 percent of

Pacific halibut are gathered in Alaskan waters and blaze solidified while still on the pontoon, so solidified fish may even be a superior alternative. Obviously, make certain to defrost solidified fish in the cooler before utilizing it appropriately.

Mediterranean One-Pan Baked Halibut

You can make this heated halibut formula any night of the week. It's easy and requires negligible cleanup (hi, sheet-container supper!) But, the key to its stunning flavor is, as it's been said, in the sauce!

Not astounding to you, the sauce is strongly Mediterranean–bunches of citrus, incredible additional virgin olive oil, new garlic, and a couple of flavors. Both the fish filets and veggies are immediately covered in this amazing sauce at that point, moved to a heating sheet. 15 minutes or so in the stove, and supper is prepared!

The sauce does its work in including incredible flavor and additionally keeping the fish soggy and delicate as it prepares.

The most effective method to Make this Halibut Recipe:

1. In the first place, we should make the sauce by blending in the ingredients in an enormous blending bowl: pizzazz and juice of 2 lemons, additional virgin olive oil, crisp garlic, seasoned salt, dark pepper, dill weed (I utilize dry), oregano and coriander.

2. Hurl the veggies in the sauce (I utilized green beans, cherry tomatoes, and onions). Use opened spoon to move the veggies to an enormous sheet pan (you'll need the remainder of the sauce for the fish)

3. Presently, do likewise and hurl the fish fillets in the sauce to cover.

4. Add fish to the sheet skillet alongside the veggies. fOn the off chance that you have any sauce left, shower all over fish and veggies

5. Prepare in 450 degrees warmed stove for around 15 minutes or something like that. In the event that you like, place the skillet under the oven for pretty much 3 minutes or something like that (I like the cherry tomatoes to pop a piece), observe cautiously. That is it, and supper is prepared!

What to Serve Along?

Since the veggies are cooked right alongside the halibut, there is no compelling reason to include more sides.Iyou like, you can serve the halibut and veggies on top of a bed of your preferred grains or, this Lebanese rice, or pasta. I like to include an enormous healthy salad like this Mediterranean Three Bean Salad, for instance. In the event that you need a canapé or starter, this avocado hummus is a decent alternative.

Remains? You can store remains in tight-cover glass holders in the refrigerator for 2 to 3 days. By and by, I like to eat remaining fish at room untimely, yet on the off chance that you need, you can warm it in a skillet over medium-low warmth just until warmed through (include a smidgen of fluid and spread quickly.)

DESCRIPTION

Make this easy halibut formula with green beans and cherry tomatoes quickly! It heats in a tasty Mediterranean-style sauce with citrus, olive oil, new garlic, and flavors.

<u>INGREDIENTS</u>

For the Sauce:

- ❖ Zest of 2 lemons
- ❖ Juice of 2 lemons
- ❖ 1 cup Private Reserve Greek additional virgin olive oil
- ❖ 1 1/2 tbsp newly minced garlic
- ❖ 2 tsp dill weed

- ❖ 1 tsp seasoned salt, more for some other time
- ❖ 1/2 tsp ground dark pepperr
- ❖ 1 tablespoon dried oregano
- ❖ 1/2 to 2/4 tablespoon ground coriander

For the Fish

- ❖ 1 lb new green beans
- ❖ 1 lb cherry tomatoes
- ❖ 1 huge yellow onion cut into half-moons
- ❖ 1 1/2 lb halibut filet, cut into 1/2-inch pieces

<u>INSTRUCTIONS</u>

1. Preheat the broiler to 425 degrees F.

2. In an enormous blending bowl, whisk the sauce ingredients together. Include the green beans, tomatoes, and onions and hurl to cover with the sauce. With a huge opened spoon or spatula, move the vegetables to a huge preparing sheet (21 x 15 x 1-inch heating sheet, for instance). Hold the vegetables to the other side or one portion of the preparing sheet and ensure they are spread out in one layer.

3. Then, add the halibut fillet strips to the rest of the sauce, hurl to cover. Move the halibut filet to the heating sheet beside the vegetables and pour any outstanding sauce on top.

4. Lightly sprinkle the halibut and vegetables with somewhat more seasoned salt.

5. Bake in 425 degrees F warmed broiler for 15 minutes. At that point, move the heating sheet to the top stove rack and sear for an additional 3 minutes or thereabouts, observing cautiously. The cherry tomatoes should start to fly under the oven.

6. When prepared, expel the heated halibut and vegetables from the stove. Present with your preferred grain, Lebanese rice, or pasta. It's a good thought to include a generous salad like this Mediterranean Three Bean Salad.

NOTES

• Cook's Tip: As with any fish, don't overcook halibut. It is prepared with its pieces effectively. Serve quickly, in the event that it sits excessively long, halibut will turn somewhat dry.

• Cook's Tip: If halibut isn't accessible to you, an alternate white fish filet will likewise work. Cod and sole are two great choices. Modify heating time, as indicated by the thickness of the fish.

• Leftover Tips: You can store remains in tight-cover glass compartments in the ice chest for 2 to 3 days. Actually, I like to eat remaining fish at room untimely, yet in the event that you need, you can warm it in a skillet over medium-low warmth just until warmed through (include a tad of fluid and spread quickly.)

Greek Chicken Souvlaki Recipe with Tzatziki {Video}

This natively constructed chicken souvlaki formula takes you to the boulevards of Athens. Make certain to see the video instructional exercise beneath.

You essentially can't go to Greece without encountering souvlaki. It's a significant Greek road food and happens to be one of my top choices.

What is the Greek Souvlaki?

Like Kabobs, the word Souvlaki basically signifies "meat on sticks." But Greeks likewise use it to depict the genuine supper—warm pita, stacked with splendidly marinated flame-broiled meat and beat with Tzatziki sauce. Different fixings are regularly included, and even a handful of fries are tucked into the pita.

Why this Greek Chicken Souvlaki Recipe works?

After a touch of research and experimentation, I've built up my own Greek chicken souvlaki formula. It's anything but a confusing formula. However, it was significant for me to hit the nail on the head.

What goes into this souvlaki formula? Three straightforward things: a wonderful Greek souvlaki marinade, quality chicken, and the pita fixings.

• Greek Souvlaki Marinade. It's a basic marinade with the ideal equalization of flavors—loads of crude garlic alongside flavors like oregano, rosemary, and sweet paprika. The fluid in this souvlaki marinade is a mix of magnificent additional virgin olive oil, lemon juice, and dry white wine. I you have the opportunity, let the chicken marinate for two or three hours or medium-term (refrigerated). Be that as it may, if not, even 30 minutes is sufficient to mix the chicken with incredible flavor.

• Pita fixings. To gather mean flame-broiled souvlaki, you need some warm Greek pita and a couple of fixings. I, as a rule, barbecue, my pita just before servings. Greek Tzatziki sauce is a MUST! And I normally include cut tomatoes, cucumbers, onions, and Kalamata olives.

What to present with Greek souvlaki?

This chicken souvlaki formula will make somewhere in the range of 10 and 12 sticks. And on the off chance that you're hoping to transform it into a Mediterranean-style BBQ party, at that point consider including a couple of salads and sides to come.

Greek salad is a characteristic expansion, yet Balela, Fattoush, Grilled Zucchini Salad and this cooling Watermelon Salad would function also. Make an enormous Mezze platter like this one, or a plate of smooth Roasted Garlic Hummus.

DESCRIPTION

Top pick chicken souvlaki formula takes you to the avenues of Athens. Best souvlaki marinade; instructions for indoor/open-air flame broiling and what to serve along.

INGREDIENTS

For Souvlaki Marinade

- ❖ 10 garlic cloves, stripped
- ❖ 2 tbsp dried oregano
- ❖ 1 tsp dried rosemary
- ❖ 1 tsp sweet paprika
- ❖ 1 tsp every Kosher salt and dark pepper
- ❖ 1/4 cup Private Reserve Greek additional virgin olive oil
- ❖ 1/4 cup dry white wine
- ❖ Juice of 1 lemon
- ❖ 2 narrows leaves

For Chicken

- ❖ 2 1/2 lb natural boneless skinless chicken bosom, fat evacuated, cut into 1/2 inch pieces

Pita Fixings

- ❖ Greek pita bread
- ❖ Tzatziki Sauce (make as indicated by this formula)
- ❖ Sliced tomato, cucumber, onions, and Kalamata olives

Thoughts for Sides to Serve Along (discretionary)

- ❖ Greek salad formula
- ❖ Roasted Garlic Hummus
- ❖ Mezze Platter
- ❖ Watermelon and Cucumber Salad

__INSTRUCTIONS__

1. Prepare the marinade. In the bowl of a little food processor, include garlic, oregano, rosemary, paprika, salt, pepper, olive oil, white wine, and lemon juice (don't include the dried sound leaves yet). Heartbeat until all-around joined.

2. Place chicken in a huge bowl and include inlet leaves. Top with marinade. Hurl to join, ensuring

chicken is well-covered with marinade. spread firmly and refrigerate for 2 hours or medium-term (see note for a faster-marinating alternative.)

3. Soak 10 to 12 wooden sticks in water for 30 to 45 minutes or something like that. Get ready Tzatziki sauce and different fixings, and in case you include Greek salad or different sides, set up those too. (a few sides like cooked garlic hummus may take longer, you can set up those ahead of time).

4. When prepared, string marinated chicken pieces through the readied sticks.

5. Prepare open-air barbecue (or iron). Brush grates with a little oil and warmth over medium-high warmth. t. Spot chicken sticks on the barbecue (or cook in groups on the iron) until very much sautéed and inside temperature registers 155° on moment read thermometer. Make certain to turn sticks equitably to cook on all sides, around 5 minutes absolute. (Change temperature of flame broil if vital). While barbecuing,

brush softly with the marinade (at that point dispose of any left marinade).

6. Transfer the chicken to serving platter and let rest for 3 minutes. In the meantime, quickly flame broil pitas and keep warm.

7. Assemble barbecued chicken souvlaki pitas. To start with, spread Tzatziki sauce on pita, include chicken pieces (take them off sticks first, obviously) at that point include veggies and olives.

8. Optional: If you need more things to add to your smorgasbord, consider Greek salad, watermelon salad, cooked garlic hummus, or a major Mezze platter.

NOTES

• Recipe notes: 1) If you don't have the opportunity, you can just marinate the chicken for 30 minutes before cooking. Simply spread and leave at room temperature. 2) Grilled Souvlaki will keep well in the ice chest for 3 days or thereabouts. Make certain to unstring the chicken from sticks, and spot in a firmly shut holder before refrigerating.

• For all the more serving thoughts: see "what to present with Greek souvlaki" up in the post.

• Recommended for this Recipe: Private Reserve Greek additional virgin olive oil (from naturally developed and prepared koroneiki olives). Spare! Attempt our Greek additional virgin olive oil group.

Best Roasted Greek Potatoes

In case you're hoping to take your broiled potato formula to the following level, I energetically prescribe attempting these Greek potatoes. Straightforward and consoling lemon cooked potatoes with new garlic. My little curve: include a sprinkle of Parmesan cheddar!

All in all, what's the key to the best Greek potatoes?

Truly, these are what you would call Greek lemon potatoes. The primary flavor creators here are lemon juice and garlic (heaps of it) — furthermore, a scramble or rosemary and paprika.

A little mystery fixing here is a sprinkle of Parmesan cheddar included halfway through preparing. This isn't really customary, yet it includes both flavor and surface.

Notes for Lemon Greek potatoes

To accomplish the perfect surface, first, the Greek potatoes are heated secured for 40 minutes or so in a lot of fluid olive oil, lemon juice, and both. As they are secured, the potatoes knead as they assimilate steam and take in the consummately seasoned fluid.

At that point, we reveal the potatoes and sprinkle Parmesan cheddar. As the Greek potatoes currently heat revealed for another 10 to 15 minutes, they completely cook as they structure a smidgen of a hull on top (as yet staying very delicate within).

DESCRIPTION

Best Greek potatoes with lemon and garlic!

INGREDIENTS

For Spice Mix

- ❖ 1 tsp seasoned salt
- ❖ 1 tsp dark pepper
- ❖ 1 tsp Sweet Paprika

- ❖ 1 tsp Organic Rosemary

For Potatoes

- ❖ 4 huge preparing potatoes, stripped, washed, cut into wedges
- ❖ 8 huge garlic cloves, cleaved
- ❖ 4 tbsp Private Reserve Greek additional virgin olive oil
- ❖ 1 lemon, juice of
- ❖ 1 1/4 cup of vegetable or chicken stock
- ❖ 1/2 cup ground Parmesan cheddar
- ❖ 1 cup parsley leaves, generally cleaved

INSTRUCTIONS

1. Preheat stove to 400 degrees F.

2. In a little bowl, combine flavors. Put in a safe spot.

3. Place potato wedges in a huge delicately oiled heating dish (I utilized this one) and sprinkle with the flavor blend. Hurl potatoes together quickly to uniformly disperse flavors.

4. In a bowl, whisk together hacked garlic, olive oil, lemon juice, and juices. Fill the heating dish with potatoes.

5. Cover the preparing dish with foil and spot in the 400 degrees F-warmed stove for 40 minutes.

6. Remove from the broiler quickly. Reveal and sprinkle Parmesan cheddar on the potato wedges. Come back to broiler revealed to broil for another 10-15 minutes or until potatoes are cooked through and have turned a decent brilliant darker with a little outside layer shaping.

7. If required, to include more shading, you may put the dish under the oven for 3 minutes or thereabouts, observing cautiously.

8. Remove from the stove. Trimming with new parsley before serving. Appreciate!

NOTES

• Recommended for this formula: all-characteristic sweet paprika; rosemary; and Private Reserve Greek additional virgin olive oil (from naturally developed and handled Koroneiki olives)

Easy Mediterranean Shrimp Recipe

This Easy shrimp formula is your pass to a tasty and speedy supper (prepared in only 25 minutes!) Here, shrimp are covered in Mediterranean flavors, at that point immediately cooked in a light white wine-olive oil sauce with shallots, chime peppers, and tomatoes. So much flavor! Serve over rice, pasta, or your preferred grain!

Take to purchasing packs of effectively stripped and deveined shrimp from the cooler area. It makes life so a lot simpler! When absolutely necessary, which happens significantly more frequently than you might suspect.

Why this Easy Shrimp Recipe Works?

In this easy shrimp formula, shrimp get enhance from a brisk covering of smoked Spanish paprika, coriander, and a spot of cayenne. Then, the shrimp are hurled in the skillet with shallots, tomato, garlic, and ringer peppers. Pulling everything together is a delectable, light sauce with a basic blend of additional virgin olive oil, white wine, and citrus.

Tips for Perfectly Cooked Shrimp

It's extremely difficult to destroy an easy shrimp formula like this one. The important thing is to maintain a strategic distance from over-cooking the shrimp. Nobody likes chewy, rubbery shrimp, isn't that so? Shrimp cook so rapidly, so don't take your eyes off the skillet. How would you realize when they're prepared?

It's truly not difficult to make sense of when shrimp are done, and their shading abandons dim to orange with brilliant red tails. At the point when you see that one side is beginning to turn pink, you are so close. By then, you may utilize your wooden spoon to hurl the shrimp snappy with the goal that it turns shading on the opposite side.

A stunt gained from is to keep eyes bolted onto the thickest piece of the shrimp (the far edge as the tail), and when the tissue at the base of the fissure where the vein was abandons translucent to dark, the shrimp is done, and you should take it off the warmth.

Recall your skillet is as yet hot regardless of whether you've killed the warmth. Shrimp will keep on cooking somewhat more.

As far as surface, superbly cooked shrimp ought to be stout and succulent, yet firm to the nibble.

Step-by-Step guidelines on How to Make This Easy Shrimp Recipe

1. Pat stripped, deveined shrimp dry and spot in a bowl. Include a little flour, flavors, salt, and pepper. Hurl to cover.

2. Attire a huge skillet (I like to utilize cast iron), soften ghee and olive oil over medium warmth. Include shallots and garlic and cook for somewhat, 2 to 3

minutes or so until fragrant (be certain not to consume the garlic.)

3. Presently include ringer peppers and cook, hurling every so often, for 4 minutes or something like that.

4. Presently include the shrimp. Cook for 1 to 2 minutes, hurling

5. Presently we include the fluid, diced tomatoes, stock, white wine, and lemon juice. Cook for 5 minutes or something like that, submerging the shrimp in with your wooden spoon. Watch for shrimp to turn brilliant orange in shading (recall, watch the shrubberies part of the shrimp when that turns to shade, shrimp is prepared.) Turn heat off and include a sprinkle of crisp parsley.

What to Serve Along?

This shrimp formula is intended to be a speedy weeknight supper, yet will absolutely dazzle organization. To transform in into supper, I commonly include a side of rice (or grain of decision) and a snappy salad to begin things off. Salad choices are interminable. In the event that you need to begin with generous salad, attempt Balela or this Mediterranean Chickpea Salad with Eggplant. Something else, this snappy 3-fixing Mediterranean salad consistently works for me.

If you have the opportunity and need to add another something to begin, this easy baba ganoush or this smoky stacked baba ganoush have been my go-tos of late.

DESCRIPTION

Easy shrimp formula, covered in Mediterranean flavors and skillet-cooked in a light white wine-olive oil sauce with shallots, chime peppers, and tomatoes. Prepared in a short time or less. Make certain to peruse the tips and look at the step-by-step photographs and video above.

INGREDIENTS

- ❖ 1 Lebanese Rice formula (or make rice as indicated by bundle), discretionary
- ❖ 1 1/4 lb enormous shrimp (or prawns), stripped and deveined (whenever solidified, make certain to defrost first)
- ❖ 1 tbsp generally useful flour
- ❖ 2 tsp smoked Spanish paprika
- ❖ 1/2 tsp each salt and pepper
- ❖ 1/2 tsp ground coriander
- ❖ 1/4 tsp cayenne
- ❖ 1/4 tsp sugar
- ❖ 1 tbsp spread (I want to utilize ghee explained margarine)
- ❖ 3 tbsp Private Reserve additional virgin olive oil
- ❖ 3 shallots (around 3 1/2 ounces), daintily cut
- ❖ 4 garlic cloves, hacked
- ❖ 1/2 green chime pepper and 1/2 yellow ringer pepper (around 6 ounces altogether), cut
- ❖ 1 cup canned diced tomato
- ❖ 1/3 cup chicken or vegetable soup

- ❖ 2 tbsp dry white wine
- ❖ 2 tbsp new lemon juice
- ❖ 1/3 cup packed parsley leaves

INSTRUCTIONS

1. First, make Lebanese rice agreeing to this formula. Leave secured and undisturbed until prepared to serve. Then again, you can make dark-colored or white rice as indicated by the locally acquired bundle.

2. Pat shrimp dry and spot it in a huge bowl. Include flour, smoked paprika, salt and pepper, coriander, cayenne, and sugar. Hurl until shrimp is well-covered.

3. In an enormous cast-iron skillet, dissolve the margarine with the olive oil over medium/medium-high warmth. Include shallots and garlic. Cook for 2-3 minutes, mixing consistently, until fragrant (be certain not to consume the garlic.) Add ringer peppers. Cook an additional 4 minutes or something like that, hurling sometimes.

4. Now include the shrimp. Cook for 1 to 2 minutes, at that point, include the diced tomatoes, soup, white wine, including lemon juice. Then, Cook it for 5 minutes or so until shrimp turns splendid orange. At long last, mix in cleaved crisp parsley.

5. Serve promptly with cooked rice

NOTES

• Cook's Tip: Shrimp cook so rapidly, so don't take your eyes off the skillet. Shrimp are prepared when their shading abandons dark to orange with splendid red tails. At the point when you see that one side is beginning to turn pink, you are so close. Utilize your wooden spoon to hurl the shrimp fast with the goal that it turns shading on the opposite side. Recall your skillet is as yet hot regardless of whether you've killed the warmth. Shrimp will keep on cooking somewhat more.

• Recommended for this formula: from our everything regular and natural zest assortments, Spanish Paprika and Ground Coriander! Private Reserve Greek additional virgin olive oil (from naturally developed and handled Greek koroneiki olives)

Skillet Garlic Dijon Chicken Recipe

Occupied cooks, make proper acquaintance with another simple, encouraging, skillet chicken formula: garlic Dijon chicken. If all else fails, it's boneless chicken thighs to the salvage! I generally keep them on hand since they are so easy to work with… and truly, kinda difficult to fail (they don't evaporate as effectively as chicken bosoms do.)

This time, to spruce up the modest chicken thighs, I made a basic sauce with new garlic, Dijon mustard, and a couple of most loved flavors. The Dijon chicken goes in my consistently utilized cast iron skillet for a speedy heat at 425 degrees Fahrenheit. The kitchen smells like paradise.

What to present with this Garlic Dijon Chicken

This garlic Dijon Chicken is a significant flexible dish that you can combine up with your preferred sides. I, for the most part, make this easy Lebanese rice and vermicelli or these Greek potatoes. Or then again, attempt these easy broiled veggies. And to light up things up, include this stacked Balela salad or my languid 3-fixing Mediterranean salad.

DESCRIPTION

Easy, enhance pressed garlic Dijon chicken is the ideal weeknight supper.

INGREDIENTS

- ❖ 1.5 lb boneless, skinless chicken thighs (6 pieces)
- ❖ Salt
- ❖ 1 enormous yellow onion, cut into huge pieces

For Garlic Dijon Sauce

- ❖ 1/3 cup Private Reserve Greek additional virgin olive oil
- ❖ 3 tsp quality Dijon Mustard
- ❖ 2 tsp quality nectar

- ❖ 6 garlic cloves, minced
- ❖ 1 tsp ground coriander
- ❖ 3/4 tsp sweet paprika
- ❖ 1/2 tsp dark pepper
- ❖ 1/2 tsp cayenne pepper (discretionary)
- ❖ pinch salt

INSTRUCTIONS

1. Preheat broiler to 425 degrees F.

2. Take back down of the refrigerator. Pat dry and season on the two sides with salt. Put in a safe spot for a couple of moments.

3. Make the nectar garlic Dijon sauce. In an enormous bowl, join olive oil, Dijon mustard, nectar, garlic, flavors, and salt. Blend.

4. Add chicken to the nectar garlic Dijon sauce. Coat each piece well with the sauce. At that point, move chicken to an enormous softly oiled cast iron skillet (or heating sheet). Pour any Dijon sauce left in a bowl on top. Include the onions.

5. Bake in a warmed stove for 25 to 30 minutes or until chicken thighs are completely cooked through (inward temperature should enroll 165 degrees F)

6. Remove from warmth and topping with new parsley. Serve hot with Lebanese Rice and stacked Balela salad or this straightforward 3-fixing Mediterranean salad (see extra recommendations above)

NOTES

• Cooking Tip: This garlic Dijon chicken heats rapidly, so it's a smart thought to get ready sides first.

• Recommended : our Private Reserve Greek additional virgin olive oil (from naturally developed and handled Koroneiki olives). And from our everything common and natural zest assortments: ground coriander, and sweet Spanish paprika.

Conventional Greek Salad Recipe

A genuinely customary Greek salad formula is intended to be of barely any ingredients—uncomplicated, very new, and absolutely tasty! And this Greek salad is all that! It's actually as served on the Greek islands and towns with ready tomatoes, cucumbers, chime peppers, onions, and velvety feta cheddar. The ideal completion is a decent sprinkle of value Greek additional virgin olive oil and a little red wine vinegar.

What goes in a conventional Greek salad Recipe?

Horiatiki, or conventional Greek salad, is served regularly from late-winter to the early piece of fall. It includes the season's quality delicious tomatoes, cucumbers, red onions, and green chime peppers. The seasoning is basic: a touch of salt and dried oregano. And the dressing is a liberal sprinkle of dazzling Greek additional virgin olive oil, and you may likewise include a little red wine vinegar.

Quality Greek kalamata olives and rich feta cheddar, produced using sheep's milk, are an absolute necessity in a customary Greek salad. And the cheddar is never disintegrated, however, served in enormous lumps or squares delegated the salad.

What doesn't go in a customary Greek salad? Here, there are no red peppers or yellow peppers. And there is no lettuce, nor some other verdant greens or vegetables in conventional Greek salad.

The way into the best Greek salad?

This present townspeople's salad is overly basic, and there isn't a deficiency of flavor. Be that as it may, it does start and end with the nature of ingredients utilized.

Pick Perfect ready tomatoes (to some degree firm yet yielding somewhat to the touch; glossy skin; fragrant);

and firm, smooth-cleaned cucumbers (I lean toward English cucumbers, which are seedless and will, in general, be better in taste). Thus, pick firm and smooth looking green chime pepper and onions.

Similarly, significant here is to ensure and dress your deliberately chosen produce with the best quality additional virgin olive oil you can discover or bear. A lower quality olive oil will be dull, or more regrettable, rotten and can demolish this straightforward salad for you.

DESCRIPTION

A really customary Greek salad formula is intended to be of hardly any ingredients: tomatoes, cucumber, green peppers, red onions, and feta cheddar. A basic dressing of phenomenal additional virgin olive oil and red wine vinegar. Meets up in a short time!

INGREDIENTS

- ❖ 4 Medium succulent tomatoes, ideally natural tomatoes
- ❖ 1 Cucumber or 3/4 English (hothouse) cucumber liked, mostly stripped making a striped example
- ❖ 1 green chime pepper, cored
- ❖ 1 medium red onion
- ❖ Greek set Kalamata olives
- ❖ Salt, a squeeze
- ❖ 4 tbsp quality additional virgin olive oil (I utilized Early Harvest Greek olive oil)
- ❖ 1–2 tbsp red wine vinegar
- ❖ Blocks of Greek feta (don't disintegrate) a great add up just as you would prefer
- ❖ 1/2 tbsp quality dried oregano

INSTRUCTIONS

1. cut the tomatoes into wedges or huge lumps (I cut a few and cut the rest in wedges).

2. Cut the mostly stripped cucumber fifty-fifty length-wise, at that point cut into thick parts (at any rate 1/2″ in thickness)

3. Thinly cut the chime pepper into rings.

4. Cut the red onion down the middle and meagerly cut into half-moons.

5. Place everything in a huge salad dish. Include a decent handful of the hollowed kalamata olives.

6. Season daintily with salt (only a squeeze).

7. Give everything an exceptionally delicate prepare to blend; don't over blend, this salad isn't intended to be handled excessively.

8. Now include the feta squares top. Sprinkle the dried oregano.

9. Serve with dried up bread!

NOTES

• Leftovers? You can refrigerate remains for 2 evenings or something like that.

• Recommended for this Recipe: Our Early Harvest Greek additional virgin olive oil (from naturally developed and handled Koroneiki olives!)

True Homemade Hummus formula

What is hummus?

Most everybody knows hummus. It's the quintessential Middle Eastern plunge made by mixing chickpeas with tahini, garlic, and citrus. Best presented with pita! And as I would like to think, no mezze is finished without a bowl of rich hummus and some warm pita.

What's in an exemplary Homemade Hummus formula?

There are four fundamental ingredients that make this hummus formula: chickpeas, tahini (sesame glue), lemon juice, and a little new garlick.

How to make hummus (the BEST additional smooth hummus)

The rundown of ingredients is short and unsurprising, not all hummus recipes are made equivalent.

It's a given, hummus kinda starts and finishes with quality chickpeas. On the off chance that you can, utilize dry chickpeas (they will require splashing medium-term, at that point cooking for 2 hours or something like that). After all other options have been exhausted, quality canned chickpeas will work (I favor natural, no-salt-included.) But to get the best, creamiest natively constructed hummus, I have 3 significant tips for you:

1. Remove the skins of the chickpeas. I don't generally do this step (for example, this broiled red pepper hummus). In any case, it truly makes a distinction. The most effortless approach to evacuate the skins is by setting cooked (or canned chickpeas) in high temp water and including around 1 ½ teaspoon of preparing pop. Let it douse for 15 minutes or something like that, at that point wash chickpeas under cool water and take the skins off.

2. Include ice blocks as hummus blend mixes. This is a stunt I gained from my relative who is an ace of the Levant kitchen. The ice 3D squares assistance in stirring the hummus into a creamier surface kinda like newly beat frozen yogurt.

DESCRIPTION

Step by step instructions to make hummus the conventional way. Straightforward. No additional flavors included. Only a plain, exemplary natively constructed hummus formula. And two or three stunts will guarantee you accomplish the best hummus ever— thick, smooth, rich, and ultra-velvety. Make certain to see the video instructional exercise too.

__INGREDIENTS__

❖ 3 cups (200 grams) cooked chickpeas, stripped (from 1 to 1/4 cup dry chickpeas or from quality canned chickpeas. See formula notes for more instructions on cooking and stripping chickpeas)

- ❖ 1 to 2 garlic cloves, minced
- ❖ 3 to 4 ice blocks
- ❖ 1/3 cup (79 grams) tahini glue
- ❖ ½ tsp fit salt
- ❖ Juice of 1 lemon
- ❖ Hot water (if necessary)
- ❖ Early Harvest Greek additional virgin olive oil
- ❖ Sumac

INSTRUCTIONS

1. Mix chickpeas with minced garlic to the bowl, Puree until a smooth, powder-like blend structure.

2. While the processor is running, include ice 3D squares, tahini, salt, and lemon juice. Mix for around 4 minutes or somewhere in the vicinity. Check, and if the consistency is excessively thick still, run the processor and gradually include a little boiling water. Mix until you arrive at a wanted smooth consistency.

3. Spread in a serving bowl and include a liberal sprinkle of Early Harvest EVOO. Add a couple of chickpeas to the center, in the event that you like.

Sprinkle sumac on top. Appreciate with warm pita wedges and your preferred veggies.

<u>NOTES</u>

1. To cook dry chickpeas: absorb chickpeas a lot of water medium-term (water should be at any rate multiplied the volume of chickpeas). At the point when prepared, channel chickpeas and spot them in a medium-sized overwhelming cooking pot. Spread with water by around 2 inches. Heat to the point of boiling, at that point, lessen warmth and stew for 1/2 to 2 hours.

2. If utilizing canned chickpeas, ensure they are depleted and flushed.

3. To strip chickpeas (cooked or from a can): spread cooked chickpeas in high temp water and include 1/2 tsp preparing pop.

4. Add 1 to 2 tablespoon of Greek yogurt to hummus to likewise include some richness, yet with this formula (and tips referenced over) this isn't required

5. Recommended for this formula: the ideal approach to complete this hummus is with a liberal shower of our astounding Early Harvest Greek additional virgin olive oil and a couple of sprinkles of sumac.

Easy Moroccan Vegetable Tagine Recipe

A straightforward vegetable tagine formula stuffed with warm Moroccan flavors. One of my new most loved one-pot suppers. Vegetarian and Gluten-free.

Consider Moroccan tagine as a succulent, gradually stewed stew. Like this Moroccan Lamb Stew, the parity of sweet and exquisite flavors, combined with the power of flavors set this vegetable tagine separated from your normal stew.

This easy Moroccan vegetable tagine starts with a couple of humble ingredients, you most likely as of now have: potatoes, carrots, onions, and garlic.

A storing bit of cleaved dried apricots is the thing that gives the unobtrusive sweetness in this healthy vegetable tagine. And to adjust it off, tart tomatoes, and a sprinkle of lemon juice (which is added at the conclusion to wake everything up).

The primary zest utilized in this easy vegetable tagine formula is another most loved in our shop: Harissa . An all-regular exceptional mix of three sorts of stew, alongside sumac, caraway, fennel, and more! To play up the profundity and warmth of harissa flavor, including a little cinnamon, coriander, and a dash of turmeric.

Generally, tagine is cooked in a dirt (or clay) pot like this one, wide at the base and bested with a restricted, cone-formed spread. Be that as it may, in this cutting edge act of spontaneity, just utilize Dutch Oven.

DESCRIPTION

Top pick vegetable tagine formula! Basic vegetable stew stuffed with the ideal parity of Moroccan flavors. Vegetarian and Gluten-free.

INGREDIENTS

- ❖ 1/4 cup Private Reserve additional virgin olive oil, more for some other time
- ❖ 2 medium yellow onions, stripped and cleaved
- ❖ 8–10 garlic cloves, stripped and cleaved
- ❖ 2 huge carrots, stripped and hacked
- ❖ 2 huge reddish-brown potatoes, stripped and cubed
- ❖ 1 huge sweet potato, stripped and cubed
- ❖ Salt
- ❖ 1 tbspHarissa flavor mix
- ❖ 1 tsp ground coriander
- ❖ 1 tsp ground cinnamon
- ❖ 1/2 tsp ground turmeric
- ❖ 2 cups canned whole stripped tomatoes
- ❖ 1/2 cup stacking hacked dried apricot
- ❖ 1 quart low-sodium vegetable stock (or soup of your decision)
- ❖ 2 cups cooked chickpeas
- ❖ 1 lemon, juice of
- ❖ Handful new parsley leaves

INSTRUCTIONS

1. In a huge overwhelming pot or Dutch Oven, heat olive oil over medium warmth until simply sparkling. Add onions and increment warmth to medium-high. Saute for 5 minutes, hurling consistently.

2. Add garlic and all the slashed veggies. Season with salt and flavors. Hurl to join.

3. Cook it for 6 to 8 minutes on medium-high warmth, blending consistently with a wooden spoon.

4. Add tomatoes, apricot, and stock. Season again with only a little run of salt.

5. Keep the warmth on medium-high, and cook for 10 minutes. At that point, decrease warmth, spread, and stew for another 20 to 25 minutes or until veggies are delicate.

6. Stir in chickpeas and cook an additional 5 minutes on low warmth.

7. Stir in lemon juice and new parsley. Taste and modify seasoning, including progressively salt or harissa zest mix exactly as you would prefer.

8. Transfer to the serving bowls and top each with a liberal shower of Private Reserve additional virgin olive oil. Serve hot with your preferred bread, couscous, or rice. Appreciate!

NOTES

• Recommended for this formula Private Reserve Greek additional virgin olive oil (from naturally developed and prepared Koroneiki olives).

• And Recommended from our Spice Collection all-regular Harissa Spice Blend, and natural ground coriander and turmeric.

Mediterranean Watermelon Salad Recipe

An easy, crisp, and very light Mediterranean watermelon salad with cucumbers, smooth feta, heaps of new herbs, and a lively nectar lime dressing! Serve it alongside other summer top picks like: barbecued chicken kabobs; Kofta; flame-broiled shrimp; salmon; flame-broiled zucchini salad; citrus avocado plunge and more.

Mediterranean Watermelon Salad Recipe

This watermelon salad begins with cubed watermelons. It's easy to strip a watermelon half and cut it up into blocks. However, you can likewise utilize a melon hotshot, in the event that you need something progressively extravagant. English cucumbers are the more extended ones, and you'll see them commonly enclosed by plastic. The explanation I love utilizing them is on the grounds that they have more slender skin that isn't waxy, and, all the more critically, they are seedless and will, in general, be better. Yet, you can utilize any cucumbers here, and you may need to strip them first.

A liberal measure of crisp herbs like mint and basil includes aroma and a punch of freshness. For a straightforward dressing, a little rancher's market nectar, lime juice, and Early Harvest Extra virgin olive oil. In all actuality, the dressing can be discretionary on the off chance that you don't want to include it, yet it brings everything together flawlessly.

No enormous "cheffy abilities" required for this formula. The way into the achievement of this watermelon salad is in picking ready watermelons. In addition to other things, a great watermelon ought to be balanced and overwhelming for its size.

A Couple Tips for this Watermelon Salad

Recall that not long after watermelons are cut, the fluid gradually leaks out of the substance, and alongside it, the sweet flavor you partner with watermelon. Along these lines, this watermelon salad is best arranged and appreciated around the same time. However, if you do need to do some preparing the prior night, or if you have a few scraps, here are two or three tips for you:

• Make-Ahead: If you have to make this watermelon salad early, you can strip and solid shape the watermelon and cucumber and set up the rest of the ingredients at that point store each in the cooler in discrete compartments. Gather the dressing and blend the salad into a single unit only a couple of moments before serving.

• Leftovers: Because this is an excessively watery salad, with watermelon and cucumber being the star ingredients, it is ideal to complete it around the same time you set it up. Nonetheless, on the off chance that you have a few scraps, you can store in a tight-top glass compartment for a night or two (test before serving.)

DESCRIPTION

An easy, new, and very light Mediterranean watermelon salad. Three primary ingredients: watermelon, cucumber, and feta cheddar. Be that as it may, to take it to the following level, we include some crisp mint, basil, and a nectar vinaigrette. The ideal dish for your next neighborhood party!

INGREDIENTS

For the Honey Vinaigrette

- ❖ 2 tbsp nectar
- ❖ 2 tbsp lime juice
- ❖ 1 to 2 tbsp quality additional virgin olive oil (I utilized Greek Early Harvest)
- ❖ pinch of salt

For the Watermelon Salad

- ❖ 1/2 watermelon, stripped, cut into 3D squares
- ❖ 1 English (or Hot House) cucumber, cubed (around 2 cupfuls of cubed cucumbers)
- ❖ 15 new mint leaves, hacked
- ❖ 15 new basil leaves, hacked
- ❖ 1/2 cup disintegrated feta cheddar, more exactly as you would prefer

INSTRUCTIONS

1. In a little bowl, whisk together the nectar, lime juice, olive oil and touch of salt. Put in a safe spot for a minute.

2. In a huge bowl or serving platter with sides, join the watermelon, cucumbers, and crisp herbs.

3. Top the watermelon salad with the nectar vinaigrette and tenderly prepare to join. Top with the feta cheddar and serve!

NOTES

• Tip for Make-Ahead: If you have to make this watermelon salad early, you can strip and solid shape the watermelon and cucumber, and set up the rest of the ingredients, at that point store each in the ice chest in isolated compartments. Gather the dressing and blend the salad into a single unit only a couple of moments before serving.

• Tips for Leftovers: Because this is an excessively watery salad, with watermelon and cucumber being the star ingredients, it is ideal to complete it around the same time you set it up. Be that as it may, if that you have a few scraps, you can store in a tight-top glass holder for a night or two (test before serving.)

• Recommended for this Recipe: Early Harvest Greek additional virgin olive oil (from naturally developed and prepared Koroneiki olives!)

Mediterranean-Style Leg of Lamb Recipe with Potatoes

In case you're hoping to make the best leg of sheep formula, this instructional exercise is all you need! Mediterranean-style leg of sheep shrouded in an exceptional rub of Mediterranean flavors, new garlic, olive oil, and lemon juice at that point broiled with potato wedges and onions. This is the ideal gala to celebrate, particularly served over a bed of Lebanese rice!

Before we bounce to the leg of sheep formula, here are a couple of tips:

• For best outcomes, buy an excellent bone-in leg of sheep. And while you're busy, request that the butcher cut back the excess off.

• Leg of sheep is as of now very delicate, and there is no compelling reason to marinate it for a significant stretch of time. In fact, in this formula, I don't marinate the leg of sheep by any means. Be that as it may, I do cover the leg of sheep with a liberal rub of garlic, Mediterranean flavors, olive oil, and lemon juice.

• Do all that you can to keep away from over-cooking it. My family enjoys a leg of sheep cooked to an ideal medium (inside temperature 140 degrees F); however, as I would like to think, it is far superior medium uncommon (interior temperature 130 degrees F). Keep in mind, since this is a major chunk of meat, there will be some fluctuation. A few sections will be pinker than others, for instance.

The Step-by-Step Instruction for this Leg of Lamb Recipe

1. To begin with, make certain to remove the sheep from the ice chest for around 45 minutes to get it closer to room temp.

2. The way into all the flavor here is the wet zest rub that goes everywhere throughout the sheep. The rub is

best arranged in a food processor. Consolidate the garlic cloves, oregano, mint, paprika, nutmeg, olive oil, and lemon juice. Mix until smooth. (In case you're making this ahead, cover and refrigerate until further notice.)

3-Before applying the rub, we give the sheep a pleasant snappy sear under the oven. At the point when the sheep are sufficiently cool to handle, we embed a couple of garlic cloves in a few cuts/openings.

3. b) Now, apply our flavor-pressed zest rub everywhere throughout the sheep. Include potatoes and onions in the simmering container (season the potatoes a piece as well.)

4. Decrease broiler warmth, and tent a bit of foil over the sheep and potatoes (you don't need the foil excessively tight). Cook for 60 minutes, at that point, evacuate the foil and meal a couple of more minutes until we arrive at wanted doneness. For a medium-ish leg of sheep, I stop when the inward temperature

registers 140 degrees F or something like that. Star tip: you can go longer on the off chance that you like. However, recall you do need to let the leg of sheep rest before serving, so it will keep on cooking through as it's resting yet.

5-As referenced when expelled from the stove, and it's critical to let the leg of sheep rest around 15 to 20 minutes before serving. This enables juices to redistribute.

How to Serve leg of sheep The Mediterranean Way?

Consistent with the Mediterranean lifestyle, this leg of sheep formula is intended to be imparted to loved ones. It is generally served family-style on one huge platter with the simmered potatoes and Lebanese rice. In the event that you have some additional dish sauce, make certain to sprinkle on top!

DESCRIPTION

Flavor-pressed Mediterranean leg of sheep formula with potatoes! Make certain to watch the video and survey the step-by-step and tips above.

INGREDIENTS

- ❖ 1 4-5 lb leg of sheep, bone-in, fat cut
- ❖ Salt and pepper
- ❖ Private Reserve additional virgin olive oil, more for some other time
- ❖ 5 garlic cloves, stripped and cut; more for some other time
- ❖ 2 cups of water
- ❖ 8 medium gold potatoes, stripped and cut into wedges
- ❖ 1 medium yellow onion, stripped and cut into wedges
- ❖ 1 tsp paprika; more for some other time
- ❖ 1 tsp garlic powder
- ❖ 1 formula Lebanese rice, discretionary
- ❖ Fresh parsley for decorating, discretionary

For the sheep rub:

- ❖ 15 garlic cloves, stripped
- ❖ 2 tbsp dried oregano
- ❖ 2 tbsp dried mint chips
- ❖ 1 tbsp paprika
- ❖ 1/2 tbsp ground nutmeg
- ❖ 1/2 cup olive oil (I utilized Private Reserve Greek additional virgin olive oil)
- ❖ 2 lemons, juice of

<u>INSTRUCTIONS</u>

1. Take the leg of sheep out of the cooler and leave in room temperature for around 60 minutes. Meanwhile, set up the rest of the ingredients and make the sheep rub.

2. In the food processor, consolidate the rub ingredients. Mix until smooth. Put in a safe spot (or in the ice chest, if getting ready ahead of time).

3. When prepared, pat the sheep dry and make a couple of cuts on the two sides. Season with salt and pepper.

4. Turn the broiler on the sear. Spot the leg of sheep on a wire rack; place the rack straightforwardly on the top stove rack with the goal that it's just a couple of inches from the oven component. Cook it for 6-8 minutes on each side until the leg of sheep is pleasantly seared. Expel from the broiler. At that point, modify the stove temperature to 375 degrees F.

5. When the sheep is sufficiently cool to handle, embed the garlic cuts in the cuts, you made before. Presently spread the leg of sheep on all sides with the wet rub you made before and placed it in a cooking container with an inside rack. Add two cups of water to the base of the cooking container.

6. Season the potato and the onion wedges with the paprika, garlic powder, and somewhat salt. At that point, include them to the container either side of the sheep.

7. Now tent an enormous bit of foil over the cooking skillet, at that point place the container on the center

rack of the 375 degrees F warmed broiler. Cook secured for 60 minutes. Expel the foil and return the cooking dish to the broiler for another 10-15 minutes or until the sheep temperature registers 140 degrees F for medium.

8. Remove the dish from the broiler and let the leg of sheep rest for in any event 20 minutes before serving.

9. If you decide to, halfway through broiling the sheep, cook the rice as per this formula.

10. Place the sheep and potatoes in a huge serving platter over a bed of Lebanese rice, in the event that you decide to. Enhancement with parsley.

11. Or, you may cut the sheep first, at that point orchestrate the cut sheep with the potatoes over the rice.

NOTES

• Pro Tip: When you buy your leg of sheep, request that the butcher cut back the excess.

• Pro Tip: Do all that you can to keep away from over-cooking it. My family enjoys leg of sheep cooked to an ideal medium (interior temperature 140 degrees F); however, as I would see it, it is far and away superior medium uncommon (inward temperature 130 degrees F). Keep in mind, since this is a major chunk of meat, there will be some changeability. A few sections will be pinker than others, for instance.

• Used in this formula: Private Reserve Greek additional virgin olive oil (from naturally developed and prepared Koroneiki olives.) And from our everything normal zest assortment: paprika and nutmeg.

Greek-Style Braised Eggplant Recipe

Top pick braised eggplant formula, arranged Greek style! Eggplants cooked to smooth delicate flawlessness with chickpeas and tomato. A splendidly fulfilling meatless supper or side dish. Low-Fat. Veggie lover.

Why this braised eggplant formula works

Since quite a while ago, cooked eggplant is a wonderful thing healthy and completely smooth. Try not to stress, by since a long time ago cooked, I don't mean a throughout the day trial (in spite of the fact that you can utilize a slow cooker here). We're discussing 45 minutes in a hot broiler.

And obviously, the eggplants are properly going with chickpeas and a decent measure of squashed tomatoes. Hacked carrots include sweetness.

Adjusting everything up here, nothing unexpected, are onions and garlic alongside cove leaf and a couple of warm flavors. All the flavor!

DESCRIPTION

Elite player braised eggplant formula arranged Greek style! Eggplants cooked to smooth delicate flawlessness with chickpeas and tomato. An impeccably fulfilling meatless supper or side dish. Low-Fat. Vegetarian. Gluten-Free.

INGREDIENTS

- 1.5 lb eggplant, cut into shapes
- Salt
- Private Reserve Greek additional virgin olive oil
- 1 enormous yellow onion, cleaved
- 1 green ringer pepper, stem and innards expelled, diced
- 1 carrot, slashed
- 6 enormous garlic cloves, minced
- 2 dry cove leaves

- ❖ 1 to 1/2 tsp sweet paprika OR smoked paprika
- ❖ 1 tsp natural ground coriander
- ❖ 1 tsp dry oregano
- ❖ 3/4 tsp ground cinnamon
- ❖ 1/2 tsp natural ground turmeric
- ❖ 1/2 tsp dark pepper
- ❖ 1 28-oz can hacked tomato
- ❖ 2 15-oz jars chickpeas, save the canning fluid
- ❖ Fresh herbs, for example, parsley and mint for decorating

INSTRUCTIONS

1. Heat broiler to 400 degrees F.

2. Place eggplant 3D squares in a colander over an enormous bowl or legitimately over your sink, and sprinkle with salt. Put in a safe spot for 20 minutes or so to enable eggplant to "work out" any harshness. Wash with water and pat dry.

3. In a huge braiser, heat 1/4 cup additional virgin olive oil over medium-high until shining yet not smoking. Include onions, peppers, and hacked carrot.

Cook for 2-3 minutes, mixing consistently, at that point include garlic, sound leaf, flavors, and a scramble of salt. Cook one more moment, mixing until fragrant.

4. Now include eggplant, hacked tomato, chickpeas, and saved chickpea fluid. Mix to join.

5. Bring to a moving bubble for 10 minutes or something like that. Mix frequently. Expel from the stovetop, spread, and move to the broiler.

6. Cook in the broiler for 45 minutes until eggplant is completely cooked through to delicate. (While eggplant is braising, make certain to check on more than one occasion to check whether progressively fluid is required. Provided that this is true, expel from stove quickly and mix in around 1/2 cup of water at once.)

7. When eggplant is prepared, expel from the stove and include a liberal sprinkle of Private Reserve EVOO, decorate with crisp herbs (parsley or mint).

NOTES

• Slow-cooker instructions: you can set up the formula up to step 3 as composed. At that point, move ingredients to your moderate cooker. Include 1 cup of water and the rest of the ingredients from step 4. Cook it on low for 4 hours or until eggplant is exceptionally delicate.

• Recommended for this formula: Private Reserve Greek additional virgin olive oil (from naturally developed and prepared Koroneiki olives). And from our everything common and natural flavor assortments: sweet paprika OR smoked paprika, coriander, and turmeric.

Kofta Kebab Recipe (with video)

This ebook is all you have to make the BEST legitimate Kofta kebab formula. Flame-broiled kofta (or kefta) are sticks of ground hamburger and sheep blended in with crisp parsley, onions, garlic, and warm Middle Eastern flavors! These kabobs will sustain a group, and there are numerous sides and salads you can serve close by (bunches of thoughts at the base of this post).

The Middle East flaunts a couple of mark foods: veggie lover well-disposed falafel; shawarma; and obviously, kabobs of different kinds, including kofta!

What is Kofta or Kefta?

We should talk kofta kebabs. The word kofta (or kefta) has its sources in Persian, and it implies grounded or beat. You can have meat kofta, seafood kofta, or even a vegan kofta.

In any case, the present kofta kebab formula is one of the more well-known dishes in Egypt–a blend of ground hamburger and sheep, mixed with onions, garlic, parsley, and a couple of my preferred Middle Eastern flavors including, allspice, cardamom, sumac, and nutmeg. Flavor paradise!

There are in excess of twelve different ways to get ready kofta kebab. This koftakabab formula is easy and genuinely valid. It is my best version of Tamimi's, and a tribute to Port Said, my Mediterranean old neighborhood.

Let me give you step-by-step that it is so easy to make kofta (Kefta), and I have a lot of thoughts underneath for what you can serve along.

Step-by-Step for this Grilled Kofta Recipe:
*Note: If you're utilizing wooden sticks, make certain to douse them for 30 minutes to 1 hour before

utilizing, so they don't get on fire.1. Hack onions garlic and parsley in the food processor.

2. Presently, include ground hamburger, sheep, bread (make a point to crush out any water out of the bread), and flavors. Run processor. Scratch sides of the processor and run again until the meat blend is all around consolidated.

3. Expel the meat blend from the food processor and spot it in an enormous bowl. Take a fistful part of the meat blend and shape it on a wooden stick. Rehash the procedure until you have come up short on meat.

3. b) Be certain each kofta kebab is around 1 inch in thickness, this is best for flame broiling. Lay the kofta kebabs on a plate fixed with material paper for the present.

4. Spot kofta kebabs on the daintily oiled, warmed gas barbecue. Flame broil over medium-high warmth for

4 minutes on one side, turn over, and barbecue for another 3-4 minutes (aggregate of 7-8 minutes.)

5. Serve the kofta kebabs promptly with pita bread, tahini, and fixings (tomato wedges, onions, more parsley) and different sides you arranged (see thoughts just beneath!)

What to Serve Along Kofta (Kefta)?

These kofta kebabs are a major group pleaser, and you can, without much of a stretch, transform them into a major Mediterranean cookout by including a couple of sides and salads. The potential outcomes of what to serve close by kofta kebabs (or kabobs) are perpetual! Here are only a couple of musings.

Salads: Fattoush; Tabouli; 3-Ingredient Mediterranean Salad; or this Fresh Tomato Salad.

Sauces and Dips: Tahini Sauce, Creamy Hummus, or Roasted Red Pepper Hummus

Sides: Mediterranean Grilled Vegetables; Spicy Skillet Potatoes (BatataHarra); Lebanese Rice; Roasted Eggplant

DESCRIPTION

An unquestionable requirement attempt genuine Kofta kebab formula: ground hamburger and sheep blended in with crisp parsley, onions, garlic, and Middle Eastern flavors. Include some Mediterranean sides and salads for your next cookout! (Thoughts and video in post above)

INGREDIENTS

- ❖ 1 medium yellow onion, quartered
- ❖ 2 garlic cloves
- ❖ 1 whole bundle parsley, stems evacuated (around 2 stuffed cups parsley leaves)
- ❖ 1 lb ground hamburger
- ❖ 1/2 lb ground sheep
- ❖ 1 cut of bread, toasted until caramelized and absorbed water until completely delicate
- ❖ Salt and pepper

- ❖ 1 1/2 tsp ground allspice
- ❖ 1/2 tsp cayenne pepper
- ❖ 1/2 tsp ground green cardamom
- ❖ 1/2 tsp ground sumac
- ❖ 1/2 tsp ground nutmeg
- ❖ 1/2 tsp paprika
- ❖ Pita bread to serve

For the Fixings:

- ❖ Tahini Sauce
- ❖ Tomato wedges
- ❖ Onion wedges
- ❖ More parsley

INSTRUCTIONS

1. Soak 10 wooden sticks in water for around 30 minutes to 60 minutes. Expel from water when you are prepared to start. Gently oil the meshes of a gas flame broil and preheat it to medium-high for around 20 minutes.

2. Prepare pita bread and fixings. I you plan to make the tahini sauce from this formula. Get ready different sides and salads before you start flame broiling.

3. In a food processor, slash the onion, garlic, and parsley.

4. Add the hamburger, sheep, bread (make certain to crush out the water totally), and the flavors. Run the processor until everything is great joined framing a pale meat blend.

5. Remove the meat blend from the food processor and spot it in an enormous bowl. Take a fistful segment of the meat blend and shape it on a wooden stick. Rehash the procedure until you have come up short on meat. For best outcomes, ensure each kofta kebab is around 1 inch in thickness.

6. Lay the speared kofta kebabs on a plate fixed with material paper

7. Place the kofta kebabs on the softly oiled, warmed gas flame broil. Flame broil on medium-high warmth for 4 minutes on one side, turn over, and barbecue for another 3-4 minutes.

8. Serve the kofta kebabs promptly with pita bread, tahini, and the fixings you arranged. See recommendations for sides and related recipes.

NOTES

• Cook's Note: For gluten-free, essentially discard the toasted bread.

• Cook's Note: If you like, you can utilize an all-hamburger or all-sheep for the kofta blend

Lebanese Rice with Vermicelli

This is a basic vegetarian rice pilaf made of three ingredients: vermicelli pasta, rice, and olive oil. Include a touch of toasted pine nuts, and you have the best side of rice! All through the Mediterranean, you will discover rice dishes like Paella; Mujadra (lentils and rice); or Hashweh (Beef and rice) that are unquestionably all the more a feast. However, this Lebanese rice with vermicelli is the consistent rice of the Middle East, and it's by a long shot the most served side dish in that piece of the world.

What is in this Lebanese Rice

Fundamental Lebanese rice ordinarily comprises broken vermicelli pasta, rice (medium or long grain rice works), and additional virgin olive oil or margarine (or a mix of both). I utilize just additional virgin olive oil here. There is nevertheless a spot of salt to season this rice.

Tips for making best Lebanese Rice

1-You should wash the rice to dispose of abundance starch, which makes rice be clingy (Lebanese rice isn't intended to be clingy). At that point, douse the rice for 2o minutes or until you can break one grain of rice by squeezing it between your pointer and your thumb. Along these lines, you abbreviate the cooking time, ensuring the inside of the grain really cooks before the outside loses its shape. Recall that the rice to use here ought not to be somewhat cooked rice.

2-To give the Lebanese rice season directly from the beginning, toast the vermicelli in olive oil until brilliant dark colored (as you'll find in the step-by-step beneath), at that point, including the rice and toast, so each rice grain is covered with the olive oil.

3-Once the rice is completely cooked, let it rest for 10-15 minutes or something like that, at that point cushion it with a fork. This again helps prevent it from getting clingy or gluey.

DESCRIPTION

Veggie lover Lebanese rice with vermicelli and pine nuts. An extraordinary side dish beside numerous Mediterranean top picks.

INGREDIENTS

- ❖ 2 cups long-grain or medium-grain rice
- ❖ Water
- ❖ 1 cup broken vermicelli pasta
- ❖ 2 1/2 tbsp olive oil
- ❖ Salt
- ❖ 1/2 cup toasted pine nuts, discretionary to wrap up

INSTRUCTIONS

1. Rinse the rice well (a couple of times) at that point, place it in a medium bowl, and spread with water. Splash for 15 to 20 minutes. Test to check whether you can without much of a stretch break a grain of rice by basically setting it between your thumb and pointer.

2. In a medium non-stick cooking pot, heat the olive oil on medium-high. Include the vermicelli and consistently mix to toast it equitably. Vermicelli should turn a pleasant brilliant darker, however, observe cautiously not to over-darker or consume it (If it consumes, you should discard the vermicelli and begin once again).

3. Add the rice and keep on blending so the rice will be well-covered with the olive oil. Season with salt.

4. Now include 3 1/2 cups of water and heat it to the point of boiling until the water altogether decreases (see the photograph below). Turn the warmth to low and cover.

5. Cook for 15-20 minutes on low. Once completely cooked, turn the warmth off and leave the rice undisturbed in its cooking pot for 10-15 minutes, at that point reveal and cushion with a fork.

6. Transfer to a serving platter and top with the toasted pine nuts. Appreciate!

NOTES

• Pro Tips: 1. You should flush the rice to dispose of abundance starch, which makes rice be clingy (Lebanese rice isn't intended to be clingy). At that point, absorb the rice a lot of water for 15-20 minutes or until you can break one grain of rice by squeezing it between your pointer and your thumb. 2.toasting the vermicelli in EVOO as an initial step is a thing that gives this extraordinary rice flavor. Try not to skirt this step. 3. On the off chance that you can look at all assistance, let the rice rest for 5 to 10 minutes before serving.

• Recommended for this formula: Private Reserve Greek additional virgin olive oil (from naturally developed and prepared Koroneiki olives).

Mediterranean Stuffed Peppers Recipe (Video and Tutorial)

Beautiful chime peppers are the ideal vessel for an assortment of stuffing alternatives. You'll cherish the Mediterranean turn this stuffed peppers formula takes! The mystery is in the rice stuffing with splendidly seasoned lean ground hamburger (or turkey), chickpeas, and crisp parsley. These healthy stuffed peppers are sans dairy and gluten-free. They can be the primary course with a side salad or wow dish for when you have an organization.

How to Make these Stuffed Peppers?

1-This formula is about the delectable Mediterranean-style rice stuffing with superbly spiced ground hamburger and chickpeas. We start by completely sautéing the meat with cleaved onions, including the chickpeas later (Yes, you can utilize ground turkey or chicken rather than hamburger). Seasoning the meat is basic, and little trace of ground allspice has a significant effect on enhancing.

2-To the meat and chickpea blend, we include rice. (I like to absorb my rice water for a couple of moments to assist it with cooking equitably and rapidly.) Continuing to include enhance, we toss in some crisp parsley, paprika, and tomato sauce. Obviously, we need fluid to cook the rice stuffing. I essentially use water. Heat to the point of boiling to decrease by 1/2 preceding turning the warmth to low. At that point, we spread and let everything cook for around 20 minutes or somewhere in the vicinity.

3-And while the rice stuffing is cooking, we prepare our brilliant chime peppers for some activity!f Obviously, If that you need to utilize only one shading, state red peppers, definitely. I like to relax the peppers a piece while including some flavor. To do that, we toss the cored peppers on the flame broil and spread for a couple of moments, turning varying to make those wonderful imprints (an indoor frying pan works similarly also.)

4-All that is left to do is stuff the perfectly scorched peppers with our completely cooked rice stuffing… at that point, prepare! To make this procedure easy and clean, snatch a heating dish and load up with around 3/4 cup water or stock. Mastermind the ringer peppers, open-side up, in the dish (the peppers can be contacting.)

At that point, spoon in the stuffing to top each pepper off (the stuffing is cooked as of now, so need to leave an excess of space for extension.) Cover firmly and prepare for 25 to 30 minutes. At that point, decorate with a little new parsley before serving.

Can these stuffed peppers be set up early?

You can deal with this stuffed pepper formula early. There are a few choices here on the off chance that you need to set up these stuffed peppers a night or two ahead of time:

1. You can full plan and cook the rice stuffing, and prep and barbecue the peppers. Store each independently in tight top compartments in the ice chest. And when prepared, stuff the peppers and adhere to heating instructions. It's ideal that you can haul the rice and peppers out of the cooler to rest at room temperature for a couple of moments before heating.

2. You can pursue the formula almost the whole way and gather the peppers in your preparing dish and stuff them. Be that as it may, don't add fluid to the preparing dish yet. Rather, spread firmly and store in cooler for as long as one night. At the point when prepared, bring to room temperature, including the fluid, and adhere to heating instructions.

Would you be able to solidify scraps?

Ifyou end up with scraps, you can solidify the stuffed peppers. To start with, make certain to cool the stuffed peppers totally. From here, you can part and store them in tight-cover glass compartments and stop for 1 to 2 months. Defrost in ice chest medium-term, and warm up in medium-warmed broiler (it includes a smidgen of fluid to your heating dish, and spread the peppers before putting in the stove.)

What to present with these Mediterranean-style stuffed peppers

For extraordinary evening gatherings, these stuffed peppers make a delightful focal point.

To serve these stuffed peppers, the primary course for a light supper, plan on 1 full pepper to 1/2 pepper for each individual. Include a side of Greek tzatziki sauce or plain Greek yogurt alongside a salad like fattoush, Greek salad, or this basic 3-fixing Mediterranean salad.

DESCRIPTION

Healthy, Mediterranean-style stuffed peppers. The mystery is in the rice stuffing with consummately spiced lean ground meat, chickpeas, and new parsley. You can even utilize ground turkey or chicken rather, on the off chance that you like. These stuffed peppers can be set up ahead. Make certain to glance through the instructional exercise and watch the video!

INGREDIENTS

- ❖ Private Reserve Greek additional virgin olive oil
- ❖ 1 little yellow onion, hacked
- ❖ 1/2 lb ground meat
- ❖ salt + pepper
- ❖ 1/2 tsp allspice
- ❖ 1/2 tsp garlic powder
- ❖ 1 cup cooked or canned chickpeas
- ❖ 1/2 cup slashed parsley, more for decorate
- ❖ 1 cup short-grain rice, absorbed water for 15 minutes, at that point depleted
- ❖ 1/2 tsp hot or sweet paprika

- ❖ 3 tbsp tomato sauce
- ❖ 2 1/4 cup water
- ❖ 6 chime peppers, any hues, tops evacuated, cored
- ❖ 3/4 cup chicken stock (or water)

INSTRUCTIONS

1. In a substantial medium pot, heat 1 tbsp of oil. Saute the slashed onions until brilliant. Presently include the meat and cook medium-high warmth, infrequently mixing, until profoundly sautéed. Mix in the chickpeas and cook quickly.

2. To a similar pot, presently include the parsley, rice, paprika, and tomato sauce; mix to consolidate. Add water and bring it to a high stew until the fluid has decreased by one half.

3. Turn the warmth to low. Spread and cook for 15-20 minutes or until the rice is completely cooked and no longer hard nor excessively chewy.

4. While cooking the rice, heat a gas flame broil to medium-high. Flame broil the chime peppers for 10-15 minutes, secured. Make certain to turn the peppers every so often with the goal that all sides get singed. Expel from the flame broil and let cool quickly.

5. Preheat the stove to 350 degrees F.

6. Assemble the chime peppers, open-side up, in a heating dish loaded up with 3/4 cup stock or water. Spoon in the cooked rice blend to stuff every one of the peppers to the extremely top.

7. Cover the preparing dish firmly with foil and spot it in the 350 degrees F warmed stove. Prepare for 20-30 minutes.

8. Remove from the broiler and embellishment with parsley, on the off chance that you like. Serve promptly with your preferred salad and a side of Greek yogurt.

NOTES

• Pro-Tip: If you're searching for a significantly more advantageous choice, substitute the lean ground meat for ground turkey or chicken.

• Cook's Tip to Prepare ahead: you can pursue the formula up to step # 3 to set up the rice. And you can likewise set up the peppers. Store each independently in tight cover holders in the ice chest. Or on the other hand, pursue the formula up to step #6 amassing the stuffed peppers in a preparing dish. In any case, don't include fluid. Rather, spread firmly and store in cooler. At the point when prepared, bring to room temperature, include fluid and heat at 350 F as trained.

• Cook's Tip for Freezing Leftovers: First, make certain to cool the stuffed peppers totally. From here, you can segment and store them in tight-top glass holders and stop for 1 to 2 months. Defrost in cooler medium-term, and warm up in medium-warmed stove (it includes a smidgen of fluid to your preparing dish, and spread the peppers before putting in the broiler.)

Easy Moroccan Lamb Stew Recipe

In case you're hoping to make the best sheep stew, this formula is all you need! Ameliorating, self-destruct delicate braised sheep with heaps of veggies, chickpeas, and warm Moroccan flavors. You can likewise make this in your slow cooker or weight cooker; instructions included for both!

Flavor-Packed Moroccan Lamb Stew

The sheep stew formula with vegetables starts with well-known healthy ingredients: onions, garlic, carrots, gold potatoes, tomatoes, chickpeas...

However, to give it that magnificent Moroccan bend, I utilize a mix of sweet and exquisite flavors–from dried organic products to a large group of warm flavors!

I realize you see those dried apricots! Utilizing dried apricots–or other dried fruits like figs or raisins–may seem like a strange decision, however, trust me, it gives

[265]

a mellow, inconspicuous sweetness to help balance the flavors in the dish without being at all overwhelming. And, if utilizing whole apricots still sounds a piece excessively daring, cleave them up into little bits utilizing a sharp blade. Mincing the apricot will assist it with bettering disintegrate in the sauce and give the flavor it needs without being excessively self-evident.

The Spicy Mixture to Flavor your Moroccan Lamb Stew

This Moroccan sheep stew utilizes a mix of various flavors and flavor-producers, for example, cinnamon, allspice, narrows leaves, and, what I consider the star zest here, Moroccan Ras el Hanout.

Ras el Hanout is a quite North African/Moroccan zest mix that incorporates notes of turmeric, cloves, ginger, cardamom, nutmeg, and more! I love it in light of its profound fragrance and the layers of warm, profound flavor it adds to dishes, particularly in something like sheep stew. You can discover Ras el Hanout here at our online shop.

A tad of Ras el Hanout goes far in this recipe.

Two Important tips for making this stew

1. What slice of Lamb to Use for Lamb Stew?

To make the ideal sheep stew, I utilize boneless leg meat contrasted with different cuts of sheep. This is a cut that is quite accessible in most markets and easy to cut up into pieces.

In spite of the fact that sheep leg is a less fatty cut of sheep, stewing (or moderate cooking in a simmering pot) separates it. And the smidgen of marbling breaks up directly in during the cooking procedure, making the sheep rich and liquefy in your mouth delicately. You can substitute leg meat in this sheep stew formula for sheep shoulder, or even substitute the sheep totally with hamburger if sheep meat isn't accessible to you.

2. Braising is the best approach!

In case you're thinking about what is the ideal approach to cook sheep stew? Braising is the place you start.

Braising begins with searing the meat before stewing it shortly of fluid. Basically, you dark-colored the meat shortly of additional virgin olive oil until you get a pleasant covering and seal in every one of the juices before cooking in your Dutch broiler (or even slow cooker) with the remainder of the ingredients and juices. Cook until the meat is pleasant and delicate.

Let me simply rehash this one tip: don't skip searing the meat, it is so easy to do and improves things greatly in creating profundity and flavor directly off the bat.

Step-by-Step for this Lamb Stew Recipe

• To make Moroccan sheep stew at home, in a huge overwhelming pot or Dutch Oven (member), saute the hacked vegetables with a little oil. I utilize Private Reserve Geek additional virgin olive oil.

• Once the vegetables mellow, expel them from the container and include the sheep with somewhat more oil if necessary. This stage, is regarded as the braising stage where you need each bit of sheep to have that firm outside layer from profound cooking that will seal in the juices, keeping the sheep delicate and soggy. The braising procedure will probably make a portion of the bits stick at the base of the pot—and that is something worth being thankful for. Any cooking adds flavor and extravagance to the sauce.

• Once the meat is dark-colored on all sides, add the vegetables back to the pot with the apricots, flavors, tomatoes, and juices. Heat everything to the point of boiling, at that point spread and move to the cook in the broiler for 1 ½ hour (check part-route through to include water if necessary.) Remove quickly from the stove, include the chickpeas, and cook another 30 to 45 minutes.

Note: Oven braising helps equitably disseminate the warmth that keeps the meat delicate and holds its deliciousness.

Sheep Stew in the Crock-Pot or Pressure Cooker

This formula is overly cordial for stewing pots and weight cookers also. Here is the manner by which you can make it in either:

To make in a stewing pot

Pursue the bearings beneath by sauteing the vegetables and sautéing the sheep. When the sheep are seared, move it into a slow cooker alongside the sauteed vegetables, apricots, flavors, tomatoes, and stock. Cook on low warmth for 6 hours. Mix in chickpeas. At that point, let cook another 1 to 2 hours (as long as

8 hours altogether.) Or cook on high for as long as 5 hours.

To make in a weight cooker.

Rather than utilizing a Dutch stove or another broiler safe cooking pot, pursue the steps beneath to saute and braise utilizing your weight cooker.

At that point, include every one of the ingredients with the exception of the chickpeas to the pot and lock the top set up — Cook for 30 minutes on high weight.

At the point when the clock is up, enable the strain to securely discharge for around 10 minutes before utilizing brisk discharge, as indicated by the manufacturer's bearings. Include the chickpeas and cook for an additional 5 minutes. Enable the strain to discharge again, as indicated by the manufacturer's instructions.

Make-Ahead and Storage Instructions

Likewise, with numerous stews, Moroccan sheep stew can be made ahead and put away in the ice chest or cooler without giving up any of the flavors.

To Make-Ahead and Refrigerate: If you're planning an evening gathering and need to work a piece ahead of time, you can make this sheep stew a day or two early and keep in the cooler. It carries it closer to room temperature before reheating in the broiler (make certain to include increasingly fluid also for reheating.) a day or two and then warmed in the stove, making an extraordinary choice for evening gatherings or getting ready for a bustling night.

Serving the Moroccan Lamb Stew

This sheep stew is really generous all alone and doesn't require much else to finish the supper. I periodically serve it with challah bread or any dried-up bread. It's additionally extraordinary, spooned over some delightful Lebanese rice or plain couscous.

DESCRIPTION

In case you're hoping to make the best sheep stew, this formula is all you need! Soothing, self-destruct delicate braised sheep with heaps of veggies, chickpeas, and warm Moroccan flavors.

Make certain to look at my tips above and watch the video for how to make this sheep stew.

INGREDIENTS

- ❖ Private Reserve Greek Extra Virgin Olive Oil
- ❖ 1 enormous yellow onion, slashed
- ❖ 3 carrots, cubed
- ❖ 6 Yukon gold potatoes (or any little potatoes), stripped, cubed
- ❖ Kosher salt and pepper
- ❖ 2.5 lb boneless leg of American sheep, fat cut, cut into shapes (Or American sheep shoulder, bones expelled, fat-cut)
- ❖ 3 huge garlic cloves, generally cleaved
- ❖ ½ cup dried apricots
- ❖ 1 cinnamon stick

- ❖ 1 inlet leaf
- ❖ 1.5 tsp ground allspice
- ❖ 1.5 tablespoon ras el hanout Moroccan flavor mix
- ❖ ½ tsp ground ginger
- ❖ 6 plum tomatoes from a can, cut in equal parts
- ❖ 2 ½ cups low-sodium meat stock
- ❖ 1 15-oz can chickpeas

INSTRUCTIONS

1. In a huge Dutch stove (offshoot) or substantial broiler-safe pot, heat 2 tbsp olive oil over medium warmth until gleaming yet not smoking.

2. In the warmed oil, saute the onions, carrots, and potatoes for 4 minutes or something like that. Include the garlic and season with salt and pepper. Expel from the pot and put aside quickly.

3. In a similar pot, include more oil if necessary, and profoundly dark-colored the sheep on all sides. Season with salt and pepper.

4. Turn warmth to medium-high and return the sauteed vegetables to the pot. Include the dried apricots, cinnamon stick narrows leaf, and flavors and mix to cover.

5. Add the plum tomatoes and stock and heat everything to the point of boiling for 5 minutes or somewhere in the vicinity.

6. Cover the pot and spot in the 350 degrees F warmed broiler for 1 ½ hour (check halfway through to include water or stock if necessary). Presently mix in the chickpeas, spread, and come back to the broiler for an additional 30 minutes.

7. Remove from the stove and serve hot with your decision of Lebanese rice, couscous, pita bread, or your preferred natural bread.

8. A straightforward Mediterranean salad like Fattoush makes an incredible starter for this generous feast.

NOTES

• Crockpot Instructions: If you like, after step #5 is finished, move the sheep stew to a huge moderate cooker embed. Spread and cook on low for around 6 hours, at that point mix in chickpeas and cook another 1 to 2 hours (aggregate of as long as 8 hours.)

• Pressure-Cooker Instructions: Instead of utilizing a Dutch broiler or another stove safe cooking pot, pursue the steps underneath to sauté and braise utilizing your weight cooker. Then, include every one of the ingredients aside from the chickpeas to the pot and lock the top set up. Cook for 30 minutes on high pressure.When the clock is up, enable the strain to securely discharge for around 10 minutes before utilizing snappy discharge as per the manufacturer's headings. Include the chickpeas and cook for an additional 5 minutes. Enable the strain to discharge again, as indicated by the manufacturer's instructions.

Mediterranean Orzo salad

Ingredients

- ❖ 1 lb. orzo
- ❖ 1/2 cup sun-dried tomatoes, diced (utilize the ones in olive oil since regardless they have dampness in them)
- ❖ 15 oz. can whole artichokes, fined diced (depleted)
- ❖ One orange ringer pepper, fined diced
- ❖ 3 green onions, finely cut
- ❖ 2 tablespoons basil, meagerly cut
- ❖ 2 oz. fragmented almonds

White Balsamic Dressing:

- ❖ 1 garlic clove, minced
- ❖ 1 tablespoon dijon mustard
- ❖ 1 tablespoon crude nectar
- ❖ 1/4 cup white balsamic vinegarr
- ❖ 13/4 cup olive oil
- ❖ Salt and pepper to taste

Instructions

1. In a little bowl, include garlic clove, dijon mustard, nectar, white balsamic, olive oil, salt, and pepper. Race to consolidate and save.

2. Heat a saute dish to medium-high warmth, include almonds and toast for 2-3 minutes. Mixing once in a while so as not to consume. Expel from the container when somewhat sautéed and place on a plate.

3. Bring an enormous pot of water to bubble. Include orzo and cook until still somewhat firm, as indicated by bundle instructions, around 8-10 minutes.

4. Drain pasta and spot in an enormous bowl, include sun-dried tomatoes, artichokes, orange chime pepper, green onions, basil, and dressing.

5. Toss to consolidate.

6. Add toasted almonds directly before serving. Hurl to consolidate and serve!

Nourishment

- ❖ Serving Size: 1/2 cup
- ❖ Calories: 209
- ❖ Sugar: 5 g
- ❖ Sodium: 71 mg
- ❖ Fat: 7 g
- ❖ Carbohydrates: 32 g
- ❖ Fiber: 4 g
- ❖ Protein: 6 g

CPSIA information can be obtained
at www.ICGtesting.com
Printed in the USA
LVHW020902301120
672997LV00004B/314